T0256108

Thieme

Pelvic Pain and Dysfunction

A Differential Diagnosis Manual

Peter A. Philip, PT, ScD, COMT, PRPC
Director of Philip Physical Therapy, LLC
New Canaan, Connecticut

79 illustrations

Thieme
Stuttgart • New York • Delhi • Rio de Janeiro

Library of Congress Cataloging-in-Publication Data

Philip, Peter A., author.

  Pelvic pain and dysfunction : a differential diagnosis manual / Peter A. Philip.

    p. ; cm.

  Includes bibliographical references and index.

  ISBN 978-3-13-173221-7 (alk. paper) – ISBN 978-3-13-173231-6 (eISBN)

  I. Title.

  [DNLM: 1. Pelvic Pain–diagnosis. 2. Chronic Pain. 3. Diagnosis, Differential. 4. Pelvic Pain–therapy. 5. Physical Therapy Modalities. WP 155]

  RC946

  617.5'5075–dc23   2014019936

© 2016 Georg Thieme Verlag KG

Thieme Publishers Stuttgart
Rüdigerstrasse 14, 70469 Stuttgart, Germany
+49 [0]711 8931 421, customerservice@thieme.de

Thieme Publishers New York
333 Seventh Avenue, New York, NY 10001 USA
+1 800 782 3488, customerservice@thieme.com

Thieme Publishers Delhi
A-12, Second Floor, Sector-2, Noida-201301
Uttar Pradesh, India
+91 120 45 566 00, customerservice@thieme.in

Thieme Publishers Rio de Janeiro, Thieme Publicações Ltda.
Edifício Rodolpho de Paoli, 25º andar
Av. Nilo Peçanha, 50 – Sala 2508,
Rio de Janeiro 20020-906 Brasil
+55 21 3172-2297 / +55 21 3172-1896

Cover design: Thieme Publishing Group
Typesetting by Thomson Digital, Noida, India

Printed in India by Manipal Technologies Ltd., Manipal 5 4 3 2 1

ISBN 978-3-13-173221-7

Also available as an e-book:
eISBN 978-3-13-173231-6

Important note: Medicine is an ever-changing science undergoing continual development. Research and clinical experience are continually expanding our knowledge, in particular our knowledge of proper treatment and drug therapy. Insofar as this book mentions any dosage or application, readers may rest assured that the authors, editors, and publishers have made every effort to ensure that such references are in accordance with **the state of knowledge at the time of production of the book.**

Nevertheless, this does not involve, imply, or express any guarantee or responsibility on the part of the publishers in respect to any dosage instructions and forms of applications stated in the book. **Every user is requested to examine carefully** the manufacturers' leaflets accompanying each drug and to check, if necessary in consultation with a physician or specialist, whether the dosage schedules mentioned therein or the contraindications stated by the manufacturers differ from the statements made in the present book. Such examination is particularly important with drugs that are either rarely used or have been newly released on the market. Every dosage schedule or every form of application used is entirely at the user's own risk and responsibility. The authors and publishers request every user to report to the publishers any discrepancies or inaccuracies noticed. If errors in this work are found after publication, errata will be posted at www.thieme.com on the product description page.

Some of the product names, patents, and registered designs referred to in this book are in fact registered trademarks or proprietary names even though specific reference to this fact is not always made in the text. Therefore, the appearance of a name without designation as proprietary is not to be construed as a representation by the publisher that it is in the public domain.

This book, including all parts thereof, is legally protected by copyright. Any use, exploitation, or commercialization outside the narrow limits set by copyright legislation, without the publisher's consent, is illegal and liable to prosecution. This applies in particular to photostat reproduction, copying, mimeographing, preparation of microfilms, and electronic data processing and storage.

Contents

Preface

It is with great pleasure that I have the opportunity to introduce to the medical community a unique means with which they can evaluate and treat the patient population suffering from pelvic maladies and pain. This textbook will draw upon my orthopedic experiences in addition to years of clinical work with, and research on, this unique patient population—those suffering with pelvic pain. It is my intention to provide the reader with an overview of the pertinent anatomy as it relates to the patient with pelvic pain, and to provide a greater understanding of the complex interactions amongst the central nervous system, peripheral nervous system, the viscera, the bony anatomy, and the musculature of the pelvis. It is with this understanding and appreciation of the complexities that the clinician will have the greatest opportunity to provide their patients the most expedient relief of their pain and distress.

Having initially studied and received two degrees in physical therapy, one a general degree and the other an orthopedic master's degree, I had never known or thought of pelvic pain as an entity, let alone would have considered evaluating the pelvic region. It was during my formative years as a young clinician that I was introduced to the concept of "pelvic pain." A patient of mine at the time was an OB/GYN. He asked me about a particular patient that he was treating without success. He asked what I thought of the patient, having given me a brief summary, and asked what I'd do to help this patient! That night I began my research into the field of pelvic pain and dysfunction, and my research continues to date.

What I found was that the evaluation and treatment strategies that I learned through my initial learning did not have the same differential diagnostic, and tissue specific, testing that I apply to my general orthopedic population of patients. In essence, when I first started in the field of pelvic pain, I was approaching the evaluation and treatments in a fashion that was less tissue specific, and more or less "press and pray," hoping that I could make the pain and muscle spasms go away.

Then there was John. John phoned the office in which I was working at the time, begging for help. He complained of progressive, excruciating pain along the head of his penis. He described his pain as being that of "26,000 knives" being "jabbed" into the head of his penis—constantly.

John was seen for an evaluation and three subsequent treatments. I did the best that I could, able to offer him transient relief, but nothing long lasting. One month later, John took his life.

It was then that I began to analyze my pelvic pain patient population through the lens of "orthopedic medicine" and the differential diagnostic concepts that are applied to determine what and where the lesion originated. Utilizing the strategies and concepts as outlined by Dr. James Cyriax and applying them to this patient population I began to see the immediate changes and improvements that I had come to expect of myself when treating the orthopedic population. It was then that I knew I had to do more research, and I began my writing. My research and writing culminated in the completion of my doctoral studies and this textbook.

To all the patients suffering, my heart goes out to you. Stay strong. Know that your body can heal. Find a capable clinician, adhere to their directives, and heal.

To the clinicians treating this patient population: be patient, be kind, and be thoughtful. Each patient is unique. Your assistance in their healthcare may in fact be lifesaving. Never underestimate the ability of the body to heal. Our role is to provide the optimal environment for healing.

May God bless you in your endeavors, and may you have great success!

Peter A. Philip, PT, ScD, COMT, PRPC

About the Author

Dr. Peter A. Philip PT, ScD, COMT, PRPC is a two-time graduate of Quinnipiac University; in 1996 with a bachelors in Physical Therapy and in 1999 with a Masters in Orthopedic Physical Therapy. In 2011, Dr. Philip completed his Doctorate of Science in Physical Therapy with a concentration in Orthopedics, Pelvic Pain and Education. Since 1997, Dr. Philip has been the owner/director of Philip Physical Therapy, which is currently located in New Canaan, Connecticut. After initiating his private practice out of his truck with a reflex hammer and folding table, he is grateful to have an office space from which to work, as driving 1,000 miles a week had become quite taxing. Treating patients with orthopedic and pelvic dysfunctions, pelvic pain, and bladder/bowel dysfunctions, he incor-porates sound differential diagnostics and treatment strategies that address the body as a functional unit, taking in a global perspective and deducing the specific pain generator involved in his patients' suffering, while also deducing the origin of the pain to best provide the patient the opportunity to prevent future pain exacerbations. In 2010, he was acknowledged by the International Association of Orthopedic Medicine (IAOM) as a leader in the field of nonsurgical medicine, and was certified as an orthopedic manual therapist (COMT). In 2014 he was one of eighteen clinicians, the only East Coast resident/clinician, and the only male in the United States of America to receive a Pelvic Rehabilitation Practitioner Certification (PRPC).

Acknowledgments

It is oft said that writing is a lonely business. Lonely for the author, who spends countless hours, days, weeks, months, and years compiling the information and distilling it into a tangible source of knowledge. Loneliness, however, is not unique to the author alone, for it is the family that bears the weight of the author's toil and work. It is in light of such unwavering support that I publicly acknowledge and state my appreciation to my wife and daughter. They, for many years, had dinners and weekends alone as I sat at my desk reading, writing, and contemplating. The time lost can never be regained, your dedication and support of me never repaid. To my wife, Fonda, I love you. You've patiently held the family together through my work, research, and writing: thank you. To my daughter, Kristianne, I love you. You are the beaming light in my life. I dedicate this book, and the knowledge within, to you.

To my parents, Peter and Willa, thank you for blessing me with the strength, fortitude, and will to persevere under dire stresses.

To my in-laws, Ded Roc and Angie, thank you for understanding my time away from your daughter during my long working days and nights. Your unyielding love and support is truly appreciated.

Dr. Russell M. Woodman: My professor, my mentor, my friend. Having met you first in 1991, you've taken me under your wing and shown me how to excel as a clinician and educator. Your wisdom, thoroughness, and dedication to perfection in the field of physical therapy are exemplary. Your assistance in helping me organize this textbook was truly an honor. Thank you.

To Uncle John Stanislaw, what would I do without your tenacious persnicketies? Without getting bogged down in a grammatical extolment, suffice to say that I appreciate your assistance in setting the standard of sapience.

To those at Thieme Publishers, whose numbers are too vast to name, I thank you. If it were not for Angelika, and her faith in me and this project, this path would never have begun. Your continued guidance and insights are appreciated. And to Torsten, having fielded many questions (many of them repeatedly) without hesitancy and with absolute professionalism, thank you.

1 Introduction to Pelvic Pain

As clinicians treating patients suffering from pelvic pain, and chronic maladies alike, we are in a unique position to offer relief and restoration of comfort and function. Our patients come to us often with the most private concerns and histories. It is imperative that we always maintain a professionally strict level of respect and privacy, knowing that these patients have often been labeled and mischaracterized by other medical practitioners and loved ones alike.

It is the intention of this text to provide an accurate, repeatable, and reliable means of deducing the cause of patients' pain, and the activities that perpetuate their dysfunction.[1,2] Multiple structures must be considered, and their interplay can't be minimized. This patient population is complex, and their symptoms often do not follow a traditional pattern of linear healing; their clinical presentation is frequently confounding. This patient population will often experience a sinusoidal healing pattern, where the ebb and flow of symptoms to the uninformed are random and unpredictable. With a greater understanding of the body's natural reaction to pain, stress, emotions, and hormonal fluctuations, our patients' healing process will be better understood.

> **Learning Objectives**
>
> - The reader will explain the necessity for physical therapy as an intervention in the patient with pelvic pain.
> - The reader will respect the delicate nature of the involved anatomy.
> - The reader will justify the concepts of differential diagnostics.
> - The reader will identify the prominent boney prominences of the innominate.

The content of this textbook focuses on pain, and in particular pelvic pain. The concepts, however, are applicable to all chronic, musculoskeletal, and urogynecologic ailments alike. This textbook discusses the evaluation and treatment of the pelvis and local genital anatomy. As such, it is imperative that the clinician maintain strict professional conduct to ensure patient comfort and modesty. When possible, drape the patient. Visualize only that which requires visualization, and only for so long as it requires visualization. Once the clinician has concluded the visual inspection of the genitals, there is often no reason to maintain an in-line view of the pelvis. Very often, the clinician will have the opportunity to sit aside the plinth, with the patient draped from the abdomen to foot, from where the clinician can conduct internal evaluation and subsequent treatments.

In maintaining and maximizing patient comfort and modesty, it is suggested that the clinician request permission each and every time visualization or contact to the genitals is to be introduced. This allows the patient to maintain control over their body, and helps ease any anxiety.

Chronic pelvic pain is defined as nonmenstrual pain localized to the pelvis that is severe enough to cause functional disability, requires medical attention, and lasts for 3 or more months. It is a confounding[3] condition or set of conditions to the patient and

physicians alike where a "negative laparoscopic examination is not synonymous with the absence of disease and does not rule out physical basis for the pain the woman is experiencing."[4] Pelvic pain may be due to visceral, somatic, or neurological disorders. Visceral disorders can initiate in the genitourinary or gastrointestinal organs. Pelvic pain can also originate in the peripheral or central nervous system. All visceral structures found within the pelvis can give rise to pelvic pain, affecting the bladder, terminal ureters, urethra, ovaries, fallopian tubes, uterus, vagina, sigmoid colon, rectum, and associated vasculature and lymphatic structures. Examples of visceral pathology are endometriosis, pelvic adhesions, ovarian masses, pelvic inflammatory disease, and irritable bowel disease. The somatic structures (fascia, musculature, ligaments, and bone) can also initiate pelvic pain, and they can refer pain to their respective dermatome. Due to the complicated nature of pelvic neuroanatomy, convergence of symptoms and cross-system expression of pain, in addition to the phenomena of central centralization and peripheralization of symptoms, have further confounded both patients and clinicians.[5,6,7]

Further complicating the patients' presentation is the frequent accompaniment of an overbearing psychosocial component, which through perseveration and activation of the periaqueductal gray and the rostroventricular mater has the capacity to expand the region of pain and increase the degree of pain experienced. Those suffering with pelvic pain undergo a barrage of psychological, sexual, and interpersonal disturbances that have been found to diminish their quality of life and will often interfere with their ability to seek a healthy, intimate relationship and may be an initiator of depression.[8,9,10,11]

Chronic pelvic pain is a frustrating condition for patients and clinicians alike[5,6,7,12,13] and accounts for 10 to 15% of all gynecologic referrals, 25 to 35% of all laparoscopies, and 10 to 15% of all hysterectomies.[4] Zondervan and colleagues state that 33% of all women will experience pelvic pain in their lifetime[14,15] and 15 to 20% of the female population age 18 to 29 years will suffer from dyspareunia,[8] whereas Sobhgol et al found the incident rate to be 54.5%.[16,17] Chronic pelvic pain, as a debilitating condition, is approaching the level of significance equivalent to that of lower back pain with regard to the interruption of work days, with 3-month prevalence in 24% of those suffering.[6,8,9] The prevalence of chronic pelvic pain among 18- to 50-year-old women is similar to that for asthma and migraine headaches.[4]

Complicating the evaluation of a patient with pelvic pain is the nature of the involved anatomy. Often too embarrassed to discuss their pain with a medical provider, those who suffer will often attempt to self-medicate and neglect their painful condition(s) for many years.[18,19]

Further confounding the medical community and complicating the formation of an accurate diagnosis and subsequent management strategy of the patient with pelvic pain is the terminology that is commonly used by the medical profession. Terms such as *vulvodynia, vaginissimus, levator ani syndrome*, and others are simply references to symptoms. These terms are as generalized as "sciatica." They do not provide the clinician or patient an indication of the origin of the symptoms or offer a direction as to possible treatment strategies.[1,2]

Physical therapy is noted as an "integral" component of a multidisciplinary approach to the treatment of pelvic pain and associated sexual dysfunctions, as musculoskeletal factors are recognized as significant contributors to the initiation and propagation of pelvic pain conditions.[20,21] A review of the current treatment literature reveals a reliance on palliative treatments that focus on the alleviation of muscle spasms through stretching (dilation therapy), massage (trigger point, Thiele's, and other), meditative/conscious relaxation (biofeedback), or surgical management (labiaectomy or pudendal nerve decompression) without consideration of the cause of the muscle spasms, nerve entrapment, or fascial restrictions.

Of interest to the clinician, and the purpose of this discussion, is the provision of a means of understanding the interrelationships of the neurological, visceral, and somatic structures and their interactions when considering the initiation and propagation of pain.

The following discussion takes into consideration the multiple possible origins of pelvic muscle spasms, hyperalgesia, and allodynia through a differential diagnostic approach that integrates the concepts of symptom reproduction, symptom elimination, embryological derivation, and neurological interactions into a model that will allow the clinician to have the opportunity to accurately determine the origin of a patient's pain and, more importantly, how to accurately and effectively eliminate the pain. Direct treatment options that consider the role of cognitive behavioral management, postural corrective exercises and postural awareness management, spinal segmental mobility and facilitation (central and peripheral sensitization), in conjunction with fascial, ligamentous, dural mobility, and referred pain patterns, are presented in a fashion that is efficient, effective, and self-manageable. This can be accomplished only through the thorough understanding of the local boney, neural, fascial, and muscular systems and the interrelationships each has with the other, the various referral patterns of each, and how to determine the origin of pain propagation to most effectively eliminate the patient's suffering.

References

[1] Cyriax J, Ed. (1982). Textbook of orthopaedic medicine. London, Philadelphia, Toronto, Sydney & Tokyo: WB Saunders & Bailliere Tindall

[2] Ombregt L, Ed. (2003). A system of orthopaedic medicine (2nd ed.). Philadelphia, London: Churchill Livingstone

[3] Karnath BM, Breitkopf DM. (2007). Acute and chronic pelvic pain in women. Retrieved September 15, 2004, from www.turner-white.com

[4] Florido J, Pérez-Lucas R, Navarrete L. Sexual behavior and findings on laparoscopy or laparotomy in women with severe chronic pelvic pain. Eur J Obstet Gynecol Reprod Biol 2008; 139: 233–236

[5] Tu FF, As-Sanie S, Steege JF. Musculoskeletal causes of chronic pelvic pain: a systematic review of diagnosis: part I. Obstet Gynecol Surv 2005a; 60: 379–385

[6] Tu FF, As-Sanie S, Steege JF. Prevalence of pelvic musculoskeletal disorders in a female chronic pelvic pain clinic. J Reprod Med 2006; 51: 185–189

[7] Tu FF, Fitzgerald CM, Kuiken T, Farrell T, Harden RN. Comparative measurement of pelvic floor pain sensitivity in chronic pelvic pain. Obstet Gynecol 2007; 110: 1244–1248

[8] Farmer MA, Meston CM. Predictors of genital pain in young women. Arch Sex Behav 2007; 36: 831–843

[9] Meston CM, Hull E, Levin RJ, Sipski M. Disorders of orgasm in women. J Sex Med 2004; 1: 66–68

[10] Pontari MA, Ruggieri MR. Mechanisms in prostatitis/chronic pelvic pain syndrome. J Urol 2004; 172: 839–845

[11] Pontari MA. Chronic prostatitis/chronic pelvic pain syndrome. Urol Clin North Am 2008; 35: 81–89, vi

[12] Steihaug S. Women's strategies for handling chronic muscle pain: a qualitative study. Scand J Prim Health Care 2007; 25: 44–48

[13] Tu FF, Fitzgerald CM, Kuiken T, Farrell T, Norman Harden R. Vaginal pressure-pain thresholds: initial validation and reliability assessment in healthy women. Clin J Pain 2008; 24: 45–50

[14] Zondervan KT, Yudkin PL, Vessey MP et al. Chronic pelvic pain in the community—symptoms, investigations, and diagnoses. Am J Obstet Gynecol 2001a; 184: 1149–1155

[15] Zondervan KT, Yudkin PL, Vessey MP et al. The community prevalence of chronic pelvic pain in women and associated illness behaviour. Br J Gen Pract 2001b; 51: 541–547

[16] Sobhgol SS, Alizadeli Charndabee SM. Rate and related factors of dyspareunia in reproductive age women: a cross-sectional study. Int J Impot Res 2007; 19: 88–94

[17] Sobhgol SS, Charandabee SM. Related factors of urge, stress, mixed urinary incontinence and overactive bladder in reproductive age women in Tabriz, Iran: a cross-sectional study. Int Urogynecol J Pelvic Floor Dysfunct 2008; 19: 367–373

[18] Lawton S, Littlewood S. (2006). Vulval skin disease: Clinical features, assessment and management. Nursing Standard (Royal College of Nursing (Great Britain): 1987), 20(42), 57–63; quiz 64

[19] Lawton S. Anatomy and function of the skin, part 1. Nurs Times 2006a; 102: 26–27

[20] Rosenbaum TY. Physiotherapy treatment of sexual pain disorders. J Sex Marital Ther 2005; 31: 329–340

[21] Rosenbaum TY. Pelvic floor involvement in male and female sexual dysfunction and the role of pelvic floor rehabilitation in treatment: a literature review. J Sex Med 2007; 4: 4–13

2 General Concepts

This chapter discusses components of differential diagnostics with which the clinician may or may not be familiar; however, they are important in the formation of a functional diagnosis that allows clinicians to better be able to treat their patients. Some of the information will be a review for the reader, whereas other information will be novel. To those for whom the information is novel: enjoy and learn. To those who "know" the information provided in this chapter, take the time to review and reflect on it and apply the concepts to your current practice.

2.1 Differential Diagnostics

So as not to "reinvent the wheel," this textbook follows the differential diagnostic and treatment concepts described by Dr. James Cyriax.

Nonsurgical, orthopedic medicine originated in England in the 1920s where an internist and orthopedic surgeon, Dr. James Cyriax, developed a system of accurately delineating a musculoskeletal diagnosis of soft-tissue musculoskeletal lesions, noting a lack of satisfactory methodology in assessing the radiotranslucent moving tissues. Dr. Cyriax realized that joints become arthritic, muscles/tendons become strained, ligaments become sprained, bursas become inflamed, nerve roots/trunks and dura mater are liable to be compressed, and joints are prone to internal derangements.

The basic principles of orthopedic medicine, according to Dr. Cyriax, are[1,2]:
- Every pain has a source.
- Treatment must reach the source.
- Treatment must benefit the source to relieve the pain.

Dr. Cyriax utilized a systematic approach that isolated the cause of pain and that lends itself to a specific diagnosis and subsequent effective treatment, based on an interpretation of positive and negative findings as they relate to applied anatomy. Active and resistive motions assess the contractile tissues and willingness to move allowing the clinician to gain an understanding of the integrity of the musculotendinous structures of the region being inspected. Passive movements are utilized during an examination to determine the integrity of noncontractile structures, ligaments, and joint surfaces. Resistance tests, otherwise known as manual muscle tests (MMT), serve a twofold function. The first is to determine the individual's capacity to initiate a muscle contraction by assessing neurological status, and the second is to determine the integrity of the muscle, tendon, and the tendinous interaction with the periosteum. In doing so, the clinician will find one of the following to be true as it relates to the patient's ability to form a muscle contraction. The contraction is:
- Strong and painless; interpretation: normal
- Strong and painful; interpretation: tendinopathy/minor breach of the muscle tendon unit
- Weak and painful; interpretation: severe musculotendinous lesion or local boney fracture
- Weak and painless; interpretation: neurological compromise or severely deconditioned

A *capsular pattern* is a term that Dr. Cyriax used to describe the presence of joint capsular changes that are associated with the normal aging process and exist in the presence of an inflammatory process. The capsular pattern is associated with a specific pattern of limitation respective to each joint. The presence of a noncapsular pattern implies that the capsule is not involved and that intra- or extraarticular tissue is inflamed or injured and is the likely source of the pain.

A critical component as it relates to the concepts of differential diagnostics revolves around the muscle spasm. Often addressed as the pathology itself, Dr. Cyriax viewed a muscle spasm as a secondary phenomenon to an affliction or injury elsewhere; a symptom, not pathology in and of itself.[1,2] Utilizing this perspective allows the treating clinician the opportunity to deduce the cause of the muscle spasm(s), and to provide the patient a tissue-specific treatment that allows the muscle spasm(s) to release, often with pain alleviation.

2.2 Reflexive Arcs

A monosynaptic reflex arc is the activation of a striated or smooth muscle that involves a single spinal cord segment. This occurs when there is an applied afferent stimulation (i.e., deep tendon reflex of the patella). This afferent stimuli synapses with a motor neuron within the ventral gray column, initiating an efferent action that terminates in the same organ in which the stimulus originated.[3,4] A disynaptic reflex arc is present when an afferent fiber enters the dorsal gray column and synapses with an association neuron that then synapses with a motor neuron within the ventral gray column. There may be modification of the motor neuron due to the input from other neurons; these neurons may be located at other levels of the spinal cord, or on the other side of the spinal cord or centrally (central nervous system [CNS]), which will allow a conscious modification of a spinal reflex.[3,4]

During the course of the evaluation of the patient with pelvic pain, the quadriceps, achilles, and bulbospongiosus reflexes will be performed to determine the neurological status of their respective nerve roots. The accurate use and interpretation of the bulbospongiosus reflex in particular is useful for the clinician in determining the cause of an asymmetrical recruitment of the pelvic floor musculature (PFM).

2.3 Embryological Derivation[1,2]

It is through an understanding of embryogenesis that the clinician will have the greatest opportunity to discover the origins, not only the perpetuator, of pain for the patient suffering with either pelvic or visceral pain. Due to the dearth of accurate clinical testing available for medical professionals with regard to patients experiencing pelvic pain, it behooves the clinician to understand the interrelationship that the various pelvic structures have with one another, and how structures from independent systems are intimately related from an embryological perspective. Utilizing this knowledge provides the clinician the opportunity to map out which visceral structures appear to be involved in the patient's condition, and by cross-testing with special tests and active motions where possible and utilizing the enclosed chart a common spinal segment or segments is often found that unites the two viscera (▶ Table 2.1). In doing

Table 2.1

Organ/Joint	C3	C4	T6	T7	T8	T9	T10	T11	T12	L1	L2	L3	L4	L5	S1	S2	S3	S4	S5	Co1	Co2
SCJ	X																				
Pancreas		X																			
Liver						X															
Gall bladder			X	X	X	X	X														
Stomach/duodenum				X	X	X	X	X	X												
Small intestine						X	X	X	X												
Epididymis							X	X													
Colon: ascending							X	X	X	X											
Kidney							X	X	X	X											
Appendix							X	X	X	X											
Ureter								X	X	X											
Bladder fundus								X	X	X											
Uterine fundus								X	X	X											
Bladder neck								X	X	X											
Vagina/penis								X	X	X											
Suprarenal gland								X	X	X											
Ovary/testes								X	X	X											
Colon; flexure											X	X									
Colon; sigmoid																	X				
Prostate																X	X	X	X		
Urethra																X	X	X	X		
Rectum																	X	X	X		

Muscle	C3	C4	T6	T7	T8	T9	T10	T11	T12	L1	L2	L3	L4	L5	S1	S2	S3	S4	S5	Co1	Co2
Upper trapezius	X	X																			
Iliopsoas									X	X	X	X	X								
Guteus: med/min													X	X	X						
Gluteus maximus														X	X						
Piriformis														X	X	X					
Obturator internus														X	X	X					
Quadratus femoris													X	X	X	X	X				
Semitendinosus													X	X	X	X	X				
Semimembranosus													X	X	X	X	X				
Adductor magnus													X	X	X	X					
Peroneus: longus, brevis & tertius													X	X	X	X	X				
Tibialis anterior													X	X	X	X					
Ext. hall. Long/brevis													X	X	X	X	X				
Triceps surae													X	X	X	X	X				
Peroneus tertius													X	X	X	X	X				

Table 2.1 (*Continued*)

Organ/Joint	C3	C4	T6	T7	T8	T9	T10	T11	T12	L1	L2	L3	L4	L5	S1	S2	S3	S4	S5	Co1	Co2
Levator ani															X	X	X	X			
Superficial transverse perineal																X	X	X			
Deep transverse perineal																X	X	X			
Bulbospongiosus															X	X	X	X			
Ischiocavernosus															X	X	X	X			
External anal sphincter															X	X	X	X			
Urethral sphincter																	X		X	X	
Coccygeus																	X	X	X	X	X

Test	C3	C4	T6	T7	T8	T9	T10	T11	T12	L1	L2	L3	L4	L5	S1	S2	S3	S4	S5	Co1	Co2
Passive scap. Apprx	T1–2																				
Abdominal reflex				X	X	X	X	X	X	X	X										
Beevor's Sign				X	X	X	X														
DTR: quadriceps											X	X									
Cremaster reflex										X	X										
Prone knee flexion										X(?)	X	X									
Clitorolabial reflex																X	X	X	X		
Bulbocavernosus reflex																X	X	X			
Straight leg raise													X	X	X	X					
DTR: achilles															X	X					
Q-tip																		X			
Pin-prick																			X		

Nerve branch:	C3	C4	T6	T7	T8	T9	T10	T11	T12	L1	L2	L3	L4	L5	S1	S2	S3	S4	S5	Co1	Co2
Superior glutea nerve													X	X	X	X					
Inferior gluteal nerve														X	X						
Lateral cutaneous branch of subcostal									X												
Lateral cutaneous branch of femoral nerve											X	X									
Genitofemoral nerve										X	X										
Ilioinguinal nerve										X	X										
Obturator nerve, cutaneous branch											X	X	X								
Medial clunial nerve															X	X	X				
Superior clunial nerve										X	X	X									

5

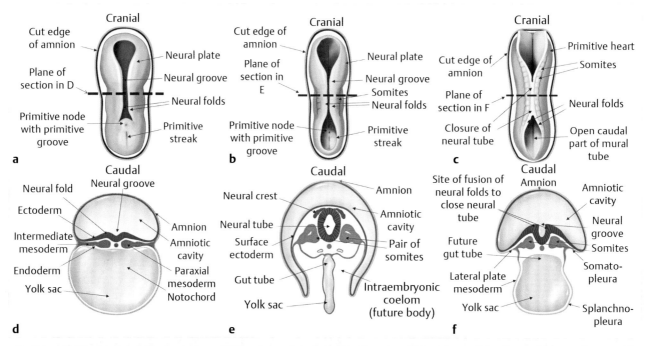

Fig. 2.1 a–f (a) Dorsal view of the neural groove. **(b)** Dorsal view of the formation of somites. **(c)** Dorsal view of the closure of the neural groove. **(d)** Transverse view of the beginning of neural crest cell migration. **(e)** Transverse view of the neural groove. **(f)** Transverse view of the neural tube, neural crest, and forming somites. (From Vacarro, Fehlings, Dvorak. Spine and Spinal Cord Trauma, Thieme Publishers: New York, 2011. Used with permission.)

so, the clinician will be able to deduce the exact spinal segment that will offer their patients immediate pain resolution, and initiate the healing process.

It is during the third week of gestation that cells of the dorsal midline of the embryo differentiate into the pseudocolumnar neuroepithelium of the neural plate from the surface ectoderm.[3] This neural plate will form the brain and spinal cord, and at the fourth week the neural plate folds dorsally and medially, eventually closing off and forming a hollow neural tube. The neural tube is a precursor to the neural canal that further differentiates into the ventricles of the brain and the central canal of the spinal cord. The lateral borders of the neural plate migrate and form the neural crest, which then further differentiates into neurons and neuroglia within the peripheral ganglia of the peripheral nervous system. The epidermis is formed from the closure of the ectoderm over the neural tube (▶ Fig. 2.1).

The caudal eminence is composed of the most caudal segment of the spinal cord that develops from specialized mesodermal structures. Secondary neurulation is the process in which the most caudal segments of the spinal cord arise from the caudal eminence, S2 to the coccygeal region. The caudal eminence further gives rise to the filum terminale, which is the anchoring attachment of the caudal end of the spinal cord.

With the closure of the neural tube, there is an elongation of the neural canal as the neuroepithelial cells elongate and retract in rhythmical fashion, which allows for the formation of the neuroblasts of the mantle layer, the precursor of the gray matter of the spinal cord, or they continue to divide as stem cells within the ventricular layer. Neuroblast differentiation continues as axon formation occurs within the neurons within the mantle layer.[3] Continued elongation and retraction produce glioblasts and neuroglial cells. Further ventricular divisions

form the ependymal cells that line the central canal of the spinal cord. Axons formation occurs as neuroblasts further differentiate into neurons. White matter of the spinal cord is a result of the axonal proliferation and elongation. Synapses are found once the axonal growth cones find their targets in the brain, spinal cord, and peripheral nerve ganglia. The gray matter further differentiates into an H-shaped column as it elongates and extends the spinal cord.

The expansion of the gray matter contains neurons that receive sensory impulses (afferent) from the sensory organs, also known as dorsal, sensory, gray columns of the spinal cord. The ventral arms of the "H" originate the motor impulses (motor) to the muscles, also known as ventral, motor gray columns of the spinal cord. The gray commissure is the area of the gray matter that connects the left and the right side of the spinal cord and is seen as the crossbar of the "H" formation. It allows for right-left and left-right communication.

Autonomic motor neurons originate at T2 to L1 and are noted as projections from either side of the "H" between the dorsal and ventral columns, the lateral gray columns. These constitute the intermediolateral gray columns of the sympathetic division of the autonomic nervous system (ANS). The sympathetic motor neurons of the sympathetic division of the ANS have two sets of components: central motor neurons that are located within the intermediolateral gray columns, and the sympathetic chain ganglia and prevertebral ganglia. The autonomic motor nervous system parasympathetic nervous system lacks the telltale gray columns; however, they can be found at S2–4, and can be classified as central motor neurons of the two motor neuron parasympathetic divisions of the ANS. The parasympathetic nervous system will also be found centrally in the hindbrain and midbrain of the brain stem, and it is due to this fact that the parasympathetic system is commonly referred to the craniosacral system.[3] Research confirms that the utilization of antibiotics, and vaccines have deleterious effects on the function of the ANS and are noted clinically as "leaky gut syndrome" and the like disrupting the function of the enteric nervous system.

The white matter of the spinal cord consists of ventral, dorsal, and lateral funiculi that transmit ascending and descending nerve impulses between different regions of the spinal cord and between the spinal cord and the brain. Blood vessels infiltrate the white matter of the spinal cord and provide the vascularization of the spinal cord. The development of the peripheral nervous system occurs as the paired somites become segmented from the paraxial mesoderm and they then interact with the neural tube, inducing a growth of the motor nerve axons from either side of the tube ventrally, the ventral/motor nerve roots. As this is occurring, the neural crest cells become detached from lateral edges of the neural plate and aggregate adjacent to the dorsolateral region of the neural tube and associate with each pair of ventral roots. These dorsal pairs differentiate into the neurons and glioblasts of the sensory dorsal root ganglia (DRG); this occurs at each level except C1. Nerve fiber projections of the DRG extend into the spinal cord and synapse with neurons in the dorsal (sensory) column. Concurrently, an outward sprouting from the DRG joins with motor fibers of the ventral root to form a spinal nerve. A dorsal root is then formed from the dorsal root ganglion and its outward growing and inward growing projections, a 31-pair spinal nerve: 8 cervical, 12 thoracic, 5 lumbar, 5 sacral ,and 1 coccygeal. *This is the theoretical model for referred pain.*[1,2,3,4] Just beyond where the spinal nerve is formed, there is another splitting; the outcome is the dorsal primary ramus and ventral primary ramus. The aforementioned rami contain the same functional makeup of axons that is present from the spinal nerves from which they originate. The dorsal ramus provides motor innervation to the true back muscles and sensory innervation to the skin over the back. It also contains sympathetic efferent and visceral afferent fibers that innervate blood vessels and glands. The ventral primary ramus provides motor innervation to the anterolateral musculature of the body wall and neck and to the upper/lower extremities. Their sensory fibers provide sensory innervation to the skin overlying these muscles and the parietal pericardium (C3 to C5), parietal pleura (T1 to T11), and parietal peritoneum (T12 to L1) of the body cavities. The ventral primary rami also contain sympathetic efferent and visceral afferent fibers.[3] With this information and understanding, the clinician will better understand the complexity of neural anatomy as it relates to the patient with pelvic pain, and will appreciate the appropriateness of performing an evaluation that is comprehensive and inclusive of the thoracic, lumbar, and sacral spines.

Clinical Note

It is through the clinical understanding and appreciation of embryological derivation, and this model of referred pain, that the clinician will have the best opportunity to gain an understanding of the patient's pain presentation

The superior aspect of the vagina, uterus, fallopian tubes, and oviducts are derived from the paramesonephric (müllerian) ducts. These ducts are common in both sexes; however, in male embryos they degenerate under the influence of antimüllerian hormone. With the absence of antimüllerian hormone, the female paramesonephric ducts continue to grow and develop, fusing at the second trimester in a distal to proximal fashion as they form the superior end of the vagina and uterus.

In female embryos, the gubernacula, embryonic structures on either side of the gonads that function to guide the terminal positioning of the gonad, form the labioscrotal folds inferiorly to the ovary superiorly. The gubernacula become attached to each paramesonephric duct and are being drawn medially as they fuse to form the vagina and uterus. This directly pulls the ovaries distally from the superior position within the posterior thoracic wall into the broad ligaments of the uterus (▶ Fig. 2.2). The two broad ligaments separate the true pelvis of females into an anterior and a posterior compartment containing the bladder and rectum, respectively. The fascia enclosed between the anterior and posterior mesothelium of the broad ligaments contains the arteries, veins, and nerves of the uterus, vagina, and ovarian ducts; the ovaries; the ovarian ligaments; and the superior ends of the round ligaments of the uterus.[3,4]

2.4 Enteric Nervous System

The enteric nervous system (ENS) is located within the wall of the gastrointestinal tract, and it shares a common embryogenesis with the brain, and it also shares common neurotransmitters including serotonin, opiates, and cholecystokinin (CCK). Under normal circumstances, the ENS automatically and independently controls motility, absorption, and secretion. Local inflammation, however, has been shown to create long-lasting and sometimes permanent changes of the ENS structures leading to functional alterations of sensory processing and motility.[3,4]

Research confirms strong interconnections between the stress response and visceral pain, acknowledging the considerable overlap within the central and peripheral nervous systems regarding the regions involved in the processing of visceral sensations and emotional regulation. Referred visceral pain can be due to alterations in the physiology of peripheral sensory neurons innervating the gut, and/or from an abnormal processing or modulation of visceral sensory information at the level of the CNS—the spinal cord, brain, or both.[5]

2.5 Behavior of Nerves

It is imperative that the clinician appreciate the typical reaction of nerves to irritation and entrapment when evaluating and treating a patient with pelvic pain and dysfunction so as to have a better means of appreciating what the patient is demonstrating and reporting, and how the patient is responding to treatment.

The reduction of radial dimensions of the peripheral nerve as a result of local entrapment will lead to pain, paresthesias, or loss of function of that nerve. Pain is due to the depolarization of free nerve endings within the investments in the target tissue connective tissues, or the dural investments of the nerve root. The degree of pain depends upon the density of nociceptive receptors within the supportive connective tissue, the intensity of compression, and where along the neuroaxis the compression is located.

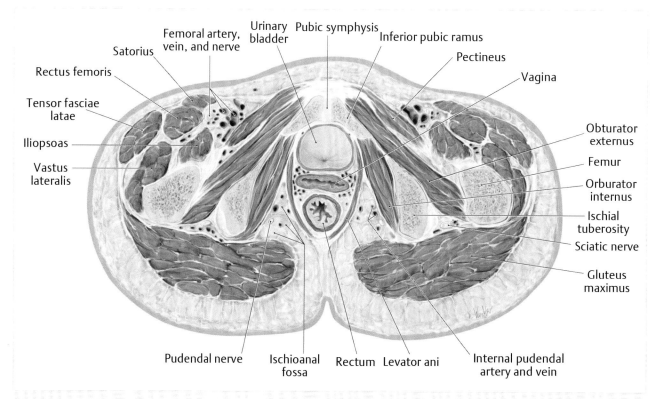

Fig. 2.2 Cross section of pelvis outlining viscera and ligaments. (From THIEME Atlas of Anatomy, General Anatomy and Musculoskeletal System, © Thieme 2005, illustration by Karl Wesker.)

Pressure upon a cutaneous nerve will present as numbness along the cutaneous region innervated by that nerve where the edges will be well defined and the center often being full of anesthesia. With continued pressure the symptoms will progress and be noted as a paresthesia ("pins-and-needles"), and finally pain. This paresthesia will be provoked by the passive movement or stroking over of the affected skin, whereas active movement does not provoke symptoms.[1,2] With continued pressure there will be an alteration along the blood–nerve barrier and this has been noted as the primary cause of nerve root dysfunction. Persistent compression will lead to atrophy of the nerve, and subsequent wallerian degeneration is likely to follow. Local edema and proliferation of connective tissue ingrowths makes recovery unlikely. Pressure on a nerve trunk will demonstrate what is known as a release phenomenon, that is, initial compression of pins-and-needles results in its subsiding to absent, only to re-present itself upon release of compression. This may be experienced as more painful paresthesia than that of the initial compression. Movement of the limb or region will provoke more pins-and-needles. Direct nerve root compression will demonstrate segmental pain *if* the dural investment is compressed and compromised. Otherwise, the nerve root is insensitive along its length. Persistent pressure will lead to pins-and-needles along its respective dermatome where the edge and aspect are poorly defined, and stroking of the skin may be provocative of pins-and-needles. Movement will not provoke pins-and-needles; however, a nerve root with impeded mobility will often be painful if the joints relative to the nerve root are taken into a motion that further stretches the nerve

root. Examples of this are noted with the straight leg raise and the prone knee flexion procedures that are performed during the evaluation. Upon tensioning of the nerve root, the clinician with a well-placed hand may be able to notice local muscle fasciculations under the palpating hand.

Learning Objectives

- The clinician will appraise the patient's symptoms and determine where along the neural axis the injury has occurred.
- The clinician will construct a treatment model that reflects the location of injury along the neural axis.

Pressure upon the dural sleeve will lead to a dermatomal reference of pain, and with persistent pressure upon the dural sleeve, eventual segmental numbness will occur due to the local necrosis of the dural sleeve. This is common with a posterolateral disk lesion. If the dura mater is compromised and infringed upon, the patient will experience what Dr. Cyriax termed *extrasegmental reference of pain*. This extrasegmental reference of pain will be experienced as an amorphic pain distribution with palpable nodules within the local musculature. These painful nodules are commonly mistaken as "trigger points," where the treatment is often directed at the alleviation of the palpable muscle nodule, whereas it should be directed at the mechanical lesion that initiated the irritation of the dura mater at the spine.

Clinical Note

When a palpable nodule is encountered, clear the spine first and observe the alleviation of the painful muscle nodule, and spasm. Remember: the lumbar spine can refer pain and muscle spasms to the perineal region!

Clinical Note

The pudendal nerve is often given responsibility for many of our patients pelvic pain. Considering that the pudendal nerve is a cutaneous nerve, the clinician must confirm that the patient initially had numbness with well-defined edges, and the center of this region being full of anesthesia. The progression of the patient's symptoms includes "pins-and-needles" and then finally pain. If the patient does not fit this pattern, then involvement of the pudendal nerve should be questioned.

2.6 Referred Pain[1,2,6]

Referred pain is the experience of "pain" that is perceived at a location different from the site of the injury; it is an error of perception by the sufferer. Various structures demonstrate unique and varying referral patterns, and the clinician needs to be aware of the presenting pattern of pain to not be misled away from the primary source of pain. A diagnosis of a patient's pain needs to be based primarily on the patient's history and clinical examination, as an accurate diagnosis is nearly impossible to make based solely on the location of the pain.[2]

Clinical Note

The clinician is to fully appreciate the various referral sources of pain as they relate to the somatic structures of the spine and viscera to best understand where the patient's pain may originate.

Possible mechanisms involved in the referral of pain may include an error at the level of the spinal cord.[2] Errors can occur at the synapses of the dorsal horns due to a convergence of information from somatic and visceral structures; as previously discussed in section 2.3, Embryological Derivation. Another source for referred pain may be a failure at the sensory cortex. To accurately approach the concept of referred pain, the clinician must constantly remember that referred pain is an error or perception. It does not indicate that pain literally "runs down" a somatic nerve.[2]

Clinical Note

Due to the infrequent sensory input of visceral structures to an individual patient's perception, as compared with input from the skin, which is common, the CNS often "mistakes" sensory information from our viscera as a cutaneous lesion.

Dr. Cyriax based his theory of referred pain on the following premises:
- Referred pain is a pain experienced elsewhere from the true site of pain.
- Skin is an organ adapted to localizing pain accurately.
- Pain is experienced in the sensory cortex, which is organized dermatome by dermatome.
- The skin is represented accurately in the sensory cortex.
- A memory storage system is located in the sensory cortex, and is fed by constant input from the skin; deeper somatic structure input is rare in the normal, healthy individual.
- A common component of referred pain is hypertonicity of the musculature through which the nerve travels.

Dr. Cyriax formulated five rules of referred pain to assist in the formulation of a diagnosis:
1. Pain radiates segmentally and does not cross midline.
2. Pain is usually felt deeply.
3. Pain is referred distally within the dermatome.
4. Pain does not necessarily cover the area of the causative lesion.
5. Pain is felt anywhere in the dermatome but not necessarily in the whole dermatome.

An overview of various referral patterns from various sources is provided in ▶ Fig. 2.3.

2.7 Connective Tissue

Epithelial tissue is typically found in sheets that are adapted to cover regions of the body and viscera. General functions of the epithelial tissue are protection, absorption, and secretion. Epithelial tissue can be found as squamous cells, more flat in nature; cuboidal cells, cube-like cells; and columnar-elongated, rectangular-shaped cells.[7]

Epithelial tissue is found in single-layered sheets of cells (simple), a multilayered sheet (stratified), or as tubular outgrowths (glands). The external surface of the body is composed of a stratified or multilayered epithelium that protects the delicate, deeper lying cells and provides insulator protection from exogenous sources.[7] Outgrowths of the epithelium form digestive glands, viscera, the tubules of the kidneys, ureters, the urinary bladder, and the urethra.

Connective tissue, unlike epithelial tissue, is more widely dispersed and separated from each other by nonliving intercellular material. Fibrous connective tissue is the most abundant tissue in the body, and it is tough and capable of withstanding torsional and traction stresses. Fibrous connective tissue may appear as a loosely woven net (skin) or as an apparently solid structure (tendons).[7]

The most common type of fiber found in connective tissue is collagen fiber, which is functionally nonelastic. In locations that are designed to allow movement, the fibers are arranged in wavy bundles (▶ Fig. 2.4). Whereas elastic fibers demonstrate the capacity to elongate and by nature are malleable they are typically outnumbered by collagen fibers. The anatomy of a healthy tendon consists of collagen bundles and extracellular matrix (ECM), where the collagen provides the tendon with tensile strength and the ECM provides structural support for

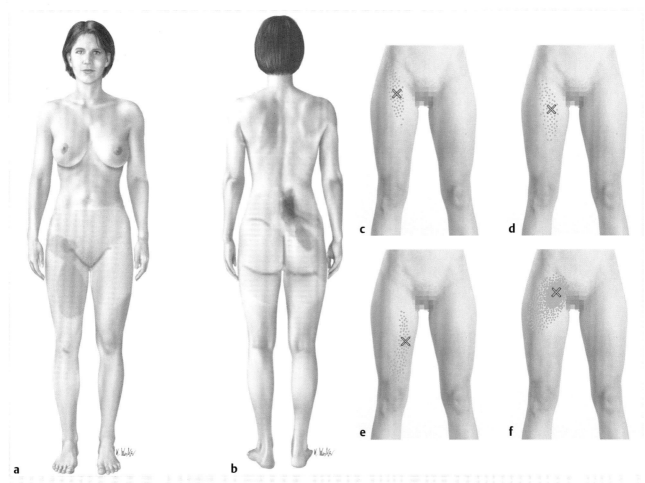

Fig. 2.3 a–f Various referral pain patterns. ([a,b] From THIEME Atlas of Anatomy, General Anatomy and Musculoskeletal System, © Thieme 2005, illustration by Karl Wesker. [c–f] From Richter P, Hebgen E. Trigger Points and Muscle Chains in Osteopathy, Thieme Publishers: Stuttgart, 2009. Used with permission.)

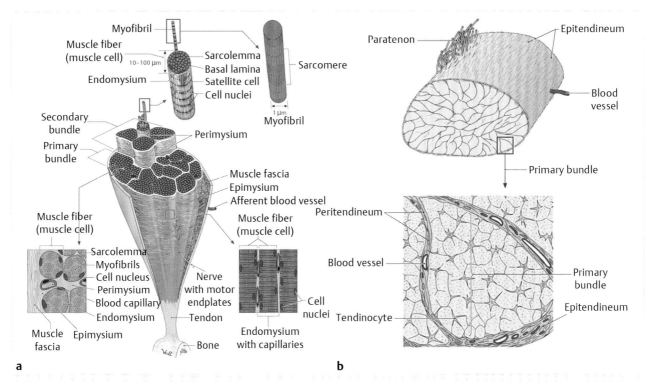

Fig. 2.4 a,b Anatomy of healthy tendon. (From THIEME Atlas of Anatomy, General Anatomy and Musculoskeletal System, © Thieme 2005, illustration by Markus Voll.)

the collagen fibers and regulates the extracellular assembly of procollagen into mature collagen.[8] Tenocytes, found among collagen fibers, are responsible for the synthesis of both the ECM and the protein procollagen building precursors. The tendon is covered by the epitenon, a sheath of fine, loose connective tissue that contains vasculature, lymphatic, and nerve supplies. The endotendon is an extension of the epitenon that runs deeper into the tendon between the tertiary bundles. Superficially, the epitenon is surrounded by paratenon: loose areolar connective tissue consisting of Type I and Type III collagen fibrils, elastic fibrils, and an inner lining of synovial cells. Collectively, the paratenon and epitenon are labeled peritendon.[8]

The myotendinous junction and the musculoskeletal junction are the regions where the muscle fibers transmit force from intracellular contractile proteins to extracellular connective tissue proteins, whereas the osteotendinous junction is where the viscoelastic tendon transmits the force to rigid bone. The former is rarely involved, whereas the latter is commonplace.

Collagens are proteins that strengthen the bones, tendons, cartilage, ligaments, vertebral disks, and skin and blood vessels of the body. Each of the tissues contains collagen with varying proportions of each collagen type: 19 collagen types have been identified; Types I, II, and III give tensile strength to tissues. Tendons also contain proteoglycans and elastin, which collectively form the ECM. Fibroblast cells are embedded in the matrix and synthesize the matrix collagen, elastin, and proteoglycans. Proteoglycans are protein/polysaccharide complexes that maintain a high water concentration that assists tendonous tissue to resist compressive forces. Proteoglycans have a pertinacious core with peripheral glycosaminoglycan that provides a gel-like cushion to compressive forces. Elastin, the elastic connective tissue of the body, is found to be interwoven with the collagen fibers to further prevent tearing.

Collagen connective tissue is classified as follows:

- Type I
  - Most abundant
  - Strong, thick fibers packed in high density
  - Located in bone, tendon, ligament, joint capsule, and annulus fibrosis
- Type II
  - Thin fibers found in articular cartilage and nucleus pulposus
- Type III
  - Most present during initial wound healing stages
  - Secures early mechanical strength
  - Thin, weak fibers are eventually replaced with Type I fibers
- Regular type
  - Ligaments, tendons, fascia, and aponeuroses are predominantly collagenous with dense and regular orientation of fibers
  - Fiber alignment dictated by stresses they experience
- Irregular type:
  - Collagen and elastin interlacing in all directions
  - Loose, extensible, and elastic and found between muscles, blood vessels, and nerves
  - Binds partly together while allowing considerable movement to take place
  - Examples: sheaths of muscles and nerves, adventitia of large blood vessels and dura mater
    - Protects against mechanical stress

Clinical Note

It is through the use of a transverse friction massage that the clinician is assisting the body in the conversion of Type III collagen to Type I collagen.

The collagen in tendons is found in a series of parallel bundles of fibers, with interspersed transverse cross links that add strength to the tendon. The typical tendon consists primarily of Type I collagen, with smaller amounts of Type III collagen. With trauma, there is destruction of local collagen. The tenocytes attempt to replenish the disturbed tissue, which results in collagen with an abnormally high Type III to Type I ratio resulting in tissue that is much more frail and friable in nature. The lesser quality collagen is seen to continue its proliferation even after the offending motion, activity, or stressor has been eliminated, indicating an alteration of function. Tissue of inferior quality often replaces damaged tissue, with the following differences:

- The total amount of collagen is decreased.
  - Breakdown exceeds repair.
- The amounts of proteoglycans and glycosaminoglycans are increased.
- The ratio of Type III to Type I collagen is abnormally high.
- The normal, parallel bundled fiber structure is disturbed.
  - The continuity of the collagen is lost with disorganized fiber structure and evidence of both collagen repair and collagen degeneration.
    - This is a key component and theoretical explanation of why transverse friction massage (TFM) works as a treatment option; it is discussed in Chapter 5.
- Microtears and collagen fiber separations are seen.
  - Collagen fibers are thin, fragile, and separated from each other.
- The number of fibroblast cells is increased.
  - Tenocytes take on unique characteristics, with a more blast-like morphology; the cells look thicker, less linear.
  - These differences show that the cells are actively trying to repair the tissue.
- The local vascularity is increased.
- Inflammatory cells are usually not seen in the tendon but sometimes are seen in the synovium and peritendinous structures, the areas around the tendon.
- Electronic microscopic observations have shown alterations in the size and shape of mitochondria in the nuclei of the tenocytes.[1,2,9,10]

Fibroblasts are cells found at intervals between the connective tissue cells and function to repair the fibers in the event of trauma.[1,3,7] Fibroblasts play a principle role in the reparative processes; during wound repair there is a migration along strands of fibrin and a distribution of elastin, collagen, and ECM. Elastin is the component that returns tissue to a relaxed state after it has been stretched.[1,3,7] Fibroblasts are responsible for creating new collagen. With tissue maturity, the activity of fibroblasts slows, and is then they are referred to as fibrocytes (tenocytes in tendons, chondrocytes in cartilage, osteocytes in bones). Fibrocytes remain inactive in their natural state, reactivating in the presence of damage and degeneration.

2.7.1 Fascia

Fascia is a dense connective tissue that plays an important role as a force transmitter in posture and movement regulation. It is composed of dense irregular connective tissue sheets in the human body; examples include:
• Aponeuroses
• Joint capsules
• Thoracolumbar-sacral fascia

> **Clinical Note**
>
> When treating a patient, minimize inflammation to prevent the fascia from tensioning, to lessen the patient's pain and more rapidly improve function.

Myofibroblasts are present in normal human fascia and found to be most dense in the lumbar fascia. A unique characteristic of myofibroblasts is that there is minimal to no activation with electrical stimulation. The introduction of inflammatory mediators such as histamine, oxcytocin, antihistaminic substance mepyramine, and cytokines, however, does lead to myofibril activation and resultant stiffness that outlasts the initial input exponentially. These myofibrils are unresponsive to epinephrine, acetylchonine, or adenosine. Maximal in vivo contractions or activation of the myofibrils result in alterations of "normal" musculoskeletal behavior.[11,12] Mechanical stretching has also been shown to activate these "connective tissue cells with muscles"; they become activated as a direct response to an applied mechanical load, functionally and locally. A positive relationship between myofibroblast activation and physical activity exists, and in part explains why in the patient that assumes the guarded and protective postures, the fascia becomes taut, that is, the adductor, transverse perineal, and pelvic floor muscles. The function of these myofibroblasts is thought be to serve as a secondary means of stabilization that does not require conscious input or direction. With injury, and persistent aggravation, however, the activation of these myofibroblasts will lead to enhanced gamma motor regulation, resulting in tissue remodeling, alterations of lumbar stability, and alterations in biomechanics. The resulting enhanced tissue tension outweighs the duration and intensity of the applied stimuli.[11,12]

Fascial properties in response to mechanical stretching:
• A 15-minutes stretch, followed by rest of 30 to 60 minutes, leads to greater resistance to stretch with follow-up stretch when compared with initial stretch.
• The greater the stretch intensity, the greater the secondary resistance to stretch.

> **Clinical Note**
>
> Treatments that attempt to treat fascia via "stretching" may in fact be the cause of persistent fascial tightness and patient pain.

The transversalis fascia is found underneath the transverse abdominis muscle and is continuous with the other layers of the deep fascia within the anterolateral abdominal wall. The subserous fascia is located deep to the transversalis fascia, and provides support to the uterine ligaments as it thickens.

The thoracolumbar fascia is a dense network of connective tissue that demonstrates connections with each muscle of the body posteriorly. It allows the spinal musculature of thoracic, lumbar, and sacral regions to function as a unit, attaching medially to all 12 thoracic vertebral spines and laterally at the angle of the ribs. In the lumbar region, the *superficial/posterior* layer separates the erector spinae muscles from latissimus dorsi muscle, medially to the spine of the lumbar and sacral vertebrae. The middle layer attaches to transverse processes of lumbar vertebrae and separates erector spinae and quadratus lumborum muscles.[3,4,13] The anterior/deep component originates on the anterior surface of the lumbar transverse processes and separates quadratus lumborum muscles from deeper psoas muscles. Transverse and internal oblique abdominals attach to an aponeurosis found along the posterior and middle layers along the lateral border and has inferior attachment to the iliolumbar ligament and iliac crest. Weakness therein predisposes an individual to intervertebral disk herniations. The thoracolumbar fascia continues through the lumbar region in three distinct layers:
• Superficial/posterior:
  ○ Separates erector spinae muscles from latissimus dorsi muscle, medially to spine of lumbar and sacral vertebrae
• Middle layer:
  ○ Attaches to transverse processes of lumbar vertebrae, separates erector spinae and quadratus lumborum
• Anterior/deep:
  ○ Anterior surface of lumbar transverse processes and separates quadratus lumborum muscles from deeper psoas muscles

Functionally, the thoracolumbar fascia assists in the transfer of forces from the lower extremity (biceps femoris to the sacrotuberous ligament (STL), to the erector spinae, to the thoracolumbar fascia) to the contralateral latissimus dorsi.

2.8 Thoracic and Lumbar Spine

The vertebrae and intervertebral disks of the thoracic, lumbar, and sacral spine are to be considered when evaluating the patient with pelvic pain. It is through these regions that the viscera-somatic innervations originate, and local restrictions have been found to propagate a patient's symptoms.[6]

Common features of the thoracic and lumbar vertebral segments include a rectangular vertebral body that is bordered on both the superior and inferior aspect by an end plate, which articulates with an intervertebral disk.

The intervertebral disk serves six purposes:
1. Increase height by adding length to the spine
2. Join vertebrae together yet allow movement
3. Equalize distribution of weight through vertebral body
4. Provide cushioning-buffering effect with trauma
5. Maintain intervertebral foramen
6. Maintain lateral facet separation

The inner portion of the intervertebral disk is known as the nucleus pulposus. It is a soft, gelatinous polysaccharide cushion between the vertebrae that exerts a uniform hydrostatic pressure upon compression. In the young it is quite distinct from the

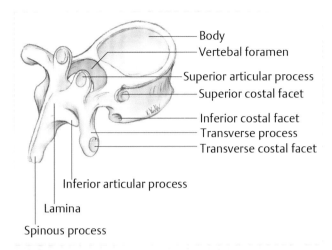

Fig. 2.5 Features of typical vertebrae. (From Fessler RG, Sekhar L. Atlas of Neurosurgical Techniques: Spine and Peripheral Nerves, Thieme Publishers: New York, 2006. Used with permission.)

annulus, whereas in the adult the separation between the two becomes less evident, less gel-like. The annulus fibrosus forms the outer shell that houses the nucleus pulposus. It is fibrocartilaginous and attaches to the vertebral end plate, the vertebral body anteriorly and posteriorly, and the longitudinal ligaments.[3,4]

Each vertebra has a vertebral arch, composed of paired pedicles and lamina, which in conjunction with the adjacent vertebra forms an intervertebral foramen, or outlet, for the spinal nerve to exit (▶ Fig. 2.5). Transverse processes extend laterally from either side of the vertebral arch, whereas the spinous process projects posteriorly. Adjacent vertebrae articulate along the superior and inferior articular processes, which are hyaline cartilage containing facet joints, and each facet joint is covered with a synovial capsule occupied with synovial fluid, forming a zygapophyseal joint (ZAJ). The synovial capsule and fluid provide lubrication to the joint. Gliding movements occur along the sliding surfaces, and are partially limited by the capacious capsule. The ZAJ is innervated by articular branches that arise from the medial branches of the posterior rami; each joint being supplied by the two adjacent nerves (▶ Fig. 2.4).

2.9 Spinal Ligaments[3,4]

Consecutive spinous processes are adjoined with membranous interspinous ligaments and stronger, more fibrous supraspinous ligaments. The interspinous ligaments connecting spinous process to spinous process from the base run posterodorsally to the apex of each process providing modest limitation to flexion. The supraspinous ligaments run the length of the spine (C7 to the sacrum) from tip to tip, merging superiorly with the nuchal ligament of the cervical spine, and they function to limit spinal flexion. Disk protrusions at L3–4, L4–5, and L5–S1 lead to tenderness of the fifth supraspinous ligament and serve as a good reminder that palpation alone does not make for a diagnosis!

Adjacent vertebral arches are united by a pale, yellow, elastic tissue referred to as the flaval ligaments. Having a near vertical disposition from the superior to adjacent inferior laminae, the flaval ligaments blend the right and left vertebral aspects at midline. These ligaments form the posterior wall of the vertebral canal, are thin cervically, and are progressively thicker through the thoracic and lumbar regions. Functionally, the flaval ligaments, with their elastic properties, resist separation of the vertebral laminae and assist in maintaining the appropriate curvatures of the vertebral column and the return from a flexed position to neutral. The interspinous and flaval ligaments possess nerves along their surface only. The sinuvertebral nerve emerges from the posterior ramus 2 mm distal to the posterior ganglion, receives branches from the sympathetic chain and loops back to the spinal canal curving upward to the base of the pedicle and running toward midline, reaching as far as the posterior longitudinal ligament (PLL) supplying the intervertebral disks, anterior and PLLs, periosteum, and dura mater (▶ Fig. 2.6).[3,14] Having two contributing branches, the most substantial of which originates from the superior intervertebral level, whereas lesser contributions originate from the two immediately inferior vertebral segments; ascending branches originate from the two layers of the PLL, the dura mater ventrally, the intervertebral disk, and the vessels of the vertebral canal; and descending branch originate from the intervertebral disk and the deeper layer of the PLL.

The PLL occupies the midline posterior to the intervertebral disk and helps prevent posterior migration of the disk. It is found within the vertebral canal posterior surface of vertebral bodies and disks, and has a superior connection to the tectorial membrane and an inferior connection to lumbar vertebrae. Its fibers fuse with the periosteum and perichondrium and taper progressively through the lumbar spine.

The anterior longitudinal ligament (ALL) runs from the occipital bone superiorly along the anterior aspect of the disks and vertebral bodies throughout the length of the spine terminating at the sacrum inferiorly. As it courses along the anterior surfaces of the vertebral bodies and disks, it blends into the periosteum and perichondrium. The intertransverse ligament consists of sheets of connective tissues that extend from one transverse process to the adjacent. They lack distinct borders and have a collagen that is less dense than a "true" ligament and are often cut during an intertransverse diskectomy.[2]

Dura mater, Latin for "tough mother," is a tough membranous tube that runs from the foramen magnum to the caudal edge of the sacral vertebrae (▶ Fig. 2.7).[2,3,4] It is composed primarily of collagen fibers, but contains a few elastin fibers, and is resistant to stretch. The purpose of the dura mater is to contain cerebral spinal fluid from the ventricles to the sacrum around the brain, spinal cord, and cauda equina—the 31 pairs of nerve roots covered by dural sheath that end at the distal edge of the intervertebral foramen. Due to the lack of elastin, dural mobility is limited, albeit notable in relationship to motion of the adjacent vertebral segments. Like the viscus, the dura mater is insensitive to cutting. It is, however, significantly sensitive to stretching. A large intraspinal space–occupying lesion such as a severe disk lesion compresses the dura mater and impedes its normal cephalic and caudal movement during neck flexion and straight leg raise testing. These moving then result in a painful stretch of the dura mater. Dural signs and symptoms that may be elicited during an evaluation are[1,2,3,4,6]:

• Pain with coughing and valsalva maneuver
• Pain with neck flexion, dura mater being 3 cm longer in flexion

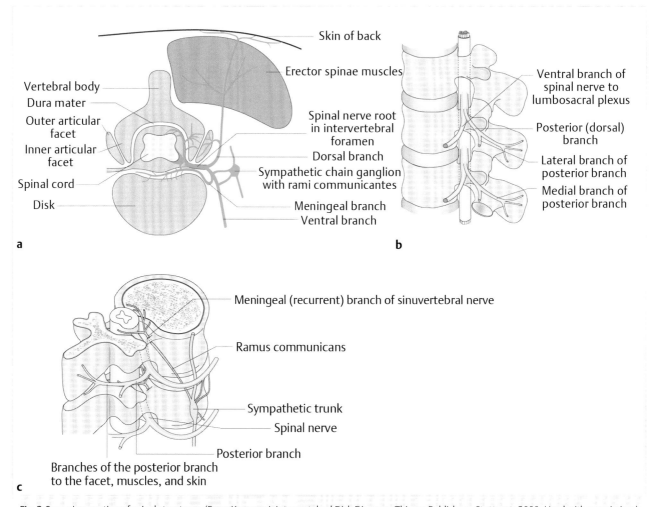

Fig. 2.6 a–c Innervation of spinal structures. (From Kraemer J. Intervertebral Disk Diseases, Thieme Publishers, Stuttgart: 2009. Used with permission.) **(a)** "Autoinnervation" of the structures of the motion segment by the meningeal branch of the spinal nerve. Sensory fibers originate mainly in the intervertebral joint, the posterior longitudinal ligament, and the spinal nerve itself. **(b)** Lumbar spinal nerve with ventral and dorsal branches (from Krämer and Nentwig, after Bogduk 1997). **(c)** The spinal nerves and their branches (from Krämer and Nentwig, after Bogduk 1997).

- Pain with dural tension testing: straight leg raising, prone knee flexion, and slump testing
- Scapular approximation, pulls the eighth and second thoracic nerves superiorly

2.10 Pelvic Osseus Anatomy

Readers are to reacquaint themselves with the relative bony anatomy of the pelvis to better understand the considerable number of structures that attach to such a confined location (▶ Fig. 2.8). It is through a strong appreciation of local bony anatomy that the clinician will be sure that specific tissues are being addressed for both diagnostic and management purposes. The skeletal pelvis is an anteriorly facing basin (pelvis by definition means basin)[7] composed of a pair of innominate bones that make up the bony component laterally, whereas the sacrum makes up the posterior aspect of the bony pelvis. Each innominate bone is formed as a union of three bones (pubis, ischium, and ilium) that are connected by cartilage in the structurally immature, but ossify in the mature adult. All three bones

contribute to the acetabulum, which articulates with the head of the femur, the coxofemoral joint. A working knowledge of the pelvic skeleton will assist in the better understanding and appreciation of the interactions of the viscera, musculature, and coxofemoral joint, and how their mechanical alignment are interrelated, with each influencing the other.

Learning Objectives

- The clinician will recall the pelvic landmarks.
- The clinician will demonstrate appropriate palpation of the pelvic landmarks.
- The clinician will appreciate the complexity and variety of muscular and ligamentous attachments to the pelvis.

The superior most bone is the ilium, which consists of three distinct components: the upper region that composed of flaring wings of bone, a lower extremity that forms the superior aspect of the acetabulum (on a clock face, the 11:00 to 2:30 position),

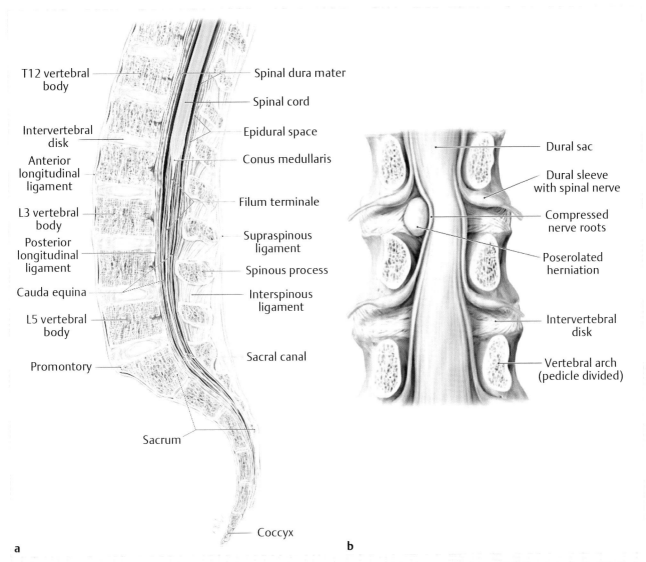

T12 vertebral body

Intervertebral disk

Anterior longitudinal ligament

L3 vertebral body

Posterior longitudinal ligament

Cauda equina

L5 vertebral body

Promontory

Sacrum

Coccyx

Spinal dura mater

Spinal cord

Epidural space

Conus medullaris

Filum terminale

Supraspinous ligament

Spinous process

Interspinous ligament

Sacral canal

Dural sac

Dural sleeve with spinal nerve

Compressed nerve roots

Poserolated herniation

Intervertebral disk

Vertebral arch (pedicle divided)

a

b

Fig. 2.7 a,b Dura mater. (From THIEME Atlas of Anatomy, General Anatomy and Musculoskeletal System, © Thieme 2005, illustration by Karl Wesker.)

and a widened iliac tuberosity posteriorly (▶ Fig. 2.9). The upper extremity of the iliac bone has three surfaces: iliac fossa, sacropelvic surface, and gluteal surface. It has a fan-shape presentation and forms the lateral prominence of the pelvis and the upper portion of the acetabulum. The iliac fossa is the anterior aspect of the ilium. It is convex in presentation and is where the iliacus muscle and a portion of the psoas muscles are found. The iliac fossa provides lateral stability to the viscera and acts as a bony attachment for the iliacus muscle. The gluteal surface has a series of ridges and indentations that provide an attachment site for the gluteal muscles. The sacropelvic surface is the region that includes the medial aspect of the iliac tuberosity and the auricular surfaces that articulate with the lateral alar surface of the sacrum. The sacroplevic surface of the iliac tuberosity provides an attachment site for the sacroiliac ligaments and the iliolumbar ligaments, and is the attachment site for the obturator internus muscle.[2,4,7] The posterior caudal portion of the ilium in conjunction with the superior posterior aspect of the ischium forms the greater sciatic notch.

The most superficial landmarks are noted in ▶ Fig. 2.10.

The Ischial bone is "V" shaped and forms the posterior-inferior portion of the pelvis, consisting of both a body and a ramus. The ischial ramus passes anteriorly and superomedially where it fuses with the inferior ramus of the pubic bone and contributes to the inferior border of the obturator foramen (▶ Fig. 2.11). The superior medial aspect of the ischium forms the inferior-posterior aspect of the acetabulum; 6:00 to 11:00. The ischial body has three distinct surfaces: femoral surface, dorsal surface, and pelvic surface. The dorsal surface includes the posterior part of the outer wall of the acetabulum, and the pelvic surface makes up a part of the lateral boundary of the ishiorectal fossa. Along the posterior border of the ischium is the lesser sciatic notch, formed from the posterior border of the body of the ischium and the posterior border of the upper extremity of the ilium.[2,4,7] The ischial tuberosity is a roughened projection that supports the weight of the body when sitting and is easily palpated just superior and anterior to the gluteal fold. The ischial spine is the most inferior-posterior aspect of

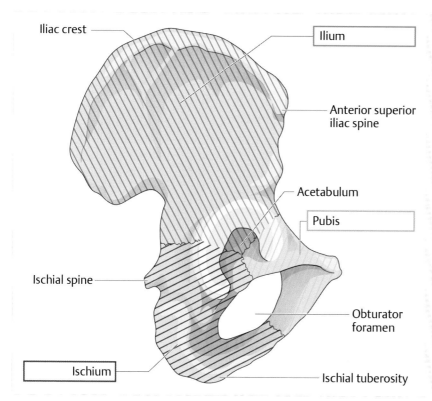

Iliac crest

Ilium

Anterior superior
iliac spine

Acetabulum

Pubis

Ischial spine

Obturator
foramen

Ischium

Ischial tuberosity

Fig. 2.8 Lateral pelvis. (From Faller A, Schuenke M. The Human Body: An Introduction to Structure and Function, Thieme Publishers, Stuttgart: 2004. Used with permission.)

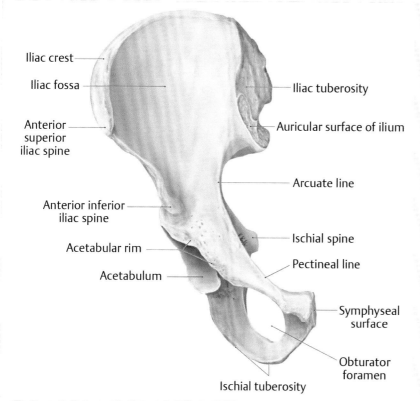

Iliac crest

Iliac fossa

Iliac tuberosity

Auricular surface of ilium

Anterior
superior
iliac spine

Arcuate line

Anterior inferior
iliac spine

Ischial spine

Acetabular rim

Pectineal line

Acetabulum

Symphyseal
surface

Obturator
foramen

Ischial tuberosity

Fig. 2.9 Anterior pelvis. (From THIEME Atlas of Anatomy, General Anatomy and Musculoskeletal System, © Thieme 2005, illustration by Karl Wesker.)

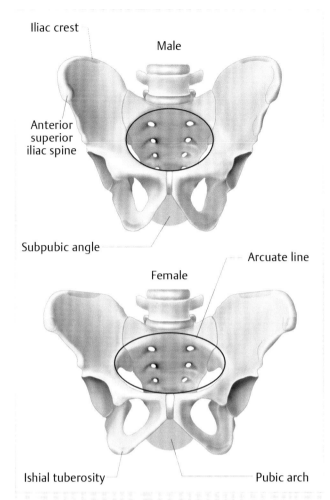

Iliac crest

Male

Anterior superior iliac spine

Subpubic angle

Arcuate line

Female

Ishial tuberosity

Pubic arch

Fig. 2.10 The male and female pelvis, anterior view. (From Reichert B. Palpation Techniques: Surface Anatomy for Physical Therapists, Thieme Publishers, Stuttgart: 2011. Used with permission.)

the bony prominence that contains multiple ridges that serve as attachments sites for the STL, the origin of the inferior gemellus muscle, the quadrates femoris muscle, and the hamstring muscles (semitendinosus, semimembranosus, and long head of biceps femoris). This inferior most extension also contains a depression that is noted as the lesser sciatic notch. The anterior aspect of the ischium extends and joins with the descending pubic ramus forming the ischiopubic ramus. The lesser sciatic notch is formed between the ischial tuberosity and the ischial spine.

Clinical Note

The obturator internus can be palpated via external means via a palpating digit being placed along the medial aspect of the ischial tuberosity, and firm pressure being applied in a cranial-lateral fashion. By doing so the clinician can glean a partial representation of the inferior-most aspect of this muscle. This may be used clinically to maintain patient modesty.

Clinical Note

The anterior SIJ ligament is a common perturbation of persistent SIJ pain and dysfunction. Often associated with palpable nodules, edema, along the external SIJ as a result of a disassociation of the sacrum and the innominate.

The pubic bone consists of three portions: body, superior ramus, and inferior ramus. The pubic bone forms the anterior aspect of the acetabulum (on a clock face, at the 2:30 to 6:00 position), and it also forms the superoventral and inferodorsal margins of the obturator foramen (▶ Fig. 2.8). The body of the pubic bones has three surfaces: ventral, dorsal, and medial. The ventral surface has an inferolateral orientation and provides an attachment site for the obturator externus muscle and the hip adductors. The dorsal surface is anterior to the urinary bladder, which is found in the anterior-inferior aspect of the abdomen; it also provides an attachment site for the pubococcygeus and the obturator internus muscles. The medial surface forms the pubic symphysis, a fibrocartilaginous joint. The superior ramus of the pubic bone provides attachment sites for the obturator externus muscle and adductors of the hip. The pubic crest is found along the superomedial prominence and provides sites for the attachment of the external obliques, internal obliques, transverse abdominis, pyramidalis, and rectus abdominis muscles. The pubic tubercles are anterolateral projections on either side of the pubic crest and are the sites for attachment of the inguinal ligaments, and attachment of the pectineus muscle at the pectineal line. The linea terminalis is formed from the pubic crest, pectin pubis, and arcuate line of the ilium. The pectin pubis provides attachment sites for the lacunar ligaments and the pectineal ligament.[2,4,7]

The pelvic rim begins at the pubic crest and continues along the pectineal line, extending to the arcuate line of the ilium and finishing at the sacrum. No muscles cross over the pelvic rim.[7]

The sacrum and coccyx are composed of fused vertebrae, each in the formation of two triangular-shaped boney elements (▶ Fig. 2.12). The cranial aspect of the first sacral vertebra articulates with the inferior aspect of the fifth lumbar vertebra, whereas the fifth sacral vertebra articulates with the first coccygeal vertebra. The sacral and coccygeal vertebrae are typically considered to fuse to one another between ages 16 and 26 years; however, this concept of the sacrum is currently being debated as the presence of sacral disks is evident on magnetic resonance imaging (MRI) and dissection alike; see photograph of a dissection of an eighty-five-year old female (▶ Fig. 2.13**a**) and MRI of a 45-year-old female (▶ Fig. 2.13**b**). The four pair of anterior sacral foramina transmit the ventral primary rami of the respective sacral spinal nerves. The coccyx is the most inferior portion of the vertebral column and consists of a fusion of the four coccgeal vertebrae. Typically it presents as a single bone; however, the first coccygeal vertebra may be separated from the distal three vertebrae. The coccygeal vertebrae are considered to be "simple" in that they have no pedicles, laminae, or spines.[2,4,7] The articulation between the auricular surface on the sacropelvic aspect of the ilium and the lateral alar mass of the sacrum is the sacroiliac joint (SIJ); it is a true synovial joint. It possesses all the characteristics of a "true joint":

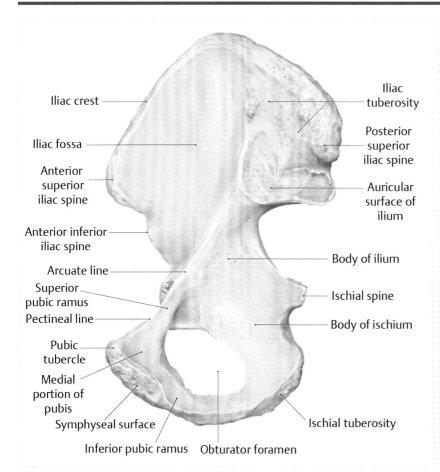

Fig. 2.11 Medial pelvis. (From THIEME Atlas of Anatomy, General Anatomy and Musculoskeletal System, © Thieme 2005, illustration by Karl Wesker.)

Iliac crest

Iliac fossa

Anterior superior iliac spine

Anterior inferior iliac spine

Arcuate line

Superior pubic ramus

Pectineal line

Pubic tubercle

Medial portion of pubis

Symphyseal surface

Inferior pubic ramus   Obturator foramen

Iliac tuberosity

Posterior superior iliac spine

Auricular surface of ilium

Body of ilium

Ischial spine

Body of ischium

Ischial tuberosity

synovial fluid, adjacent bones having ligamentous connections, cartilaginous surfaces permitting movement, and a fibrous joint capsule with a synovial lining. The articular capsule of the joint is buried within three strong ligaments: the ventral or anterior sacroiliac ligament that spans the vertical length of the SIJ, the interosseous sacroiliac ligament that fills in the spaces between the sacrum and iliac bones, and the dorsal sacroiliac ligament that covers the posterior aspect of the SIJ. Friction within the SIJ along the two articular surfaces is related to the degree of macroscopic roughening on the articular surfaces; both surfaces have ridges and grooves that increase their friction coefficients. These are more present in men than in women, suggesting greater mobility in the female SIJ then their male counterparts. Functionally, the SIJ transmits loading forces from the spine to the lower extremity, and vice versa. The center of gravity in women is more posterior to that of males, increasing rotational forces in the female SIJ (▶ Fig. 2.14).[3] The resultant quandary for women as a result of the greater mobility of the SIJ and the fact that their center of gravity is more posterior than their male counterparts is that their collective PFM is subject to greater stabilization stresses and strains in providing the dynamic stability required for locomotion and visceral homeostasis.

Clinical Note

The anterior aspect of the SIJ is innervated by L4-S3 anteriorly, and L2-S2 posteriorly, while that of the pubic symphysis is innervated by S3-5 posteriorly, and L2-L4 anteriorly.

The female pelvis is not considered completely developed until the age of 25 to 30 years of age, thus rendering the female more susceptible to avulsion injuries.[7,9,10,15,16] See ▶ Fig. 2.15, which demonstrates the average age of complete union at the epiphyses of the pelvis.[7]

Clinical Note

During the course of the history, the clinician is to ask about physical activities that the patient had partaken in during their youth and young adulthood as a means of determining the possibility of undocumented avulsion injuries.

Pelvic avulsion injuries occur in both the young and the active mature person; however, they are more common in the skeletally immature population. Typically, avulsion injuries occur as a result of a single violent movement or a combination of lower-load microtraumas at the unfused apophysis at the level of the tendonous insertion, analagous to a common musculotendinous injury in the skeletally mature. Avulsion injuries to the pelvis are common in the skeletally immature due to the inherent weakness along the unfused apophysis, and result in a separation and retraction of the partially ossified apophysis.[17,18] Apophyseal injures typically result from a violent, forceful contraction of the respective muscle, and is commonly associated with jumping, sprinting, or running.

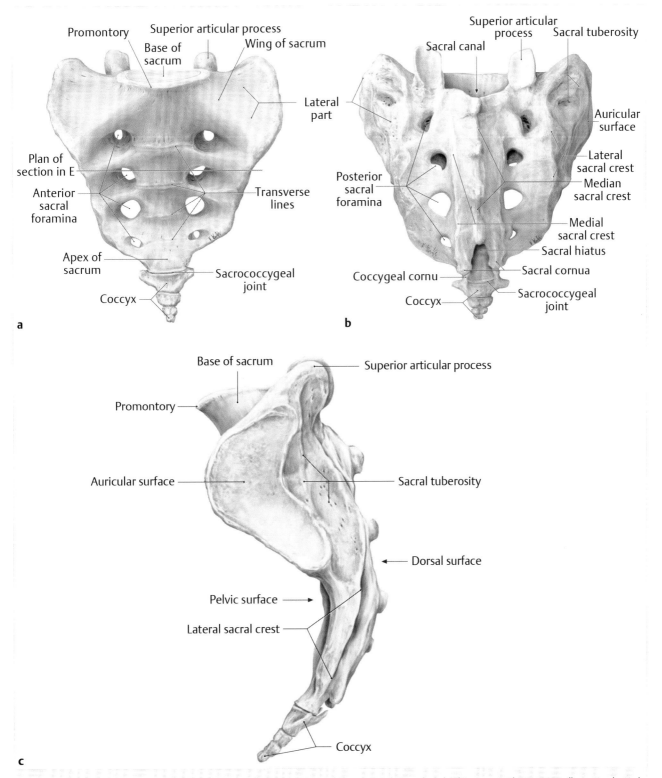

Fig. 2.12 **a–c** Sacrum and coccyx. (From THIEME Atlas of Anatomy, General Anatomy and Musculoskeletal System, © Thieme 2005, illustration by Karl Wesker.)

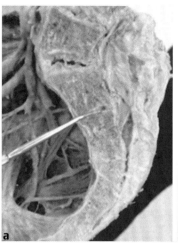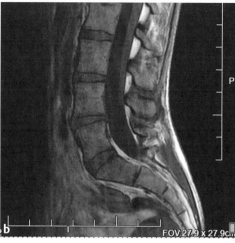

Fig. 2.13 a,b Sacral disks.

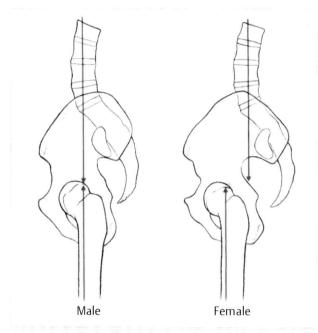

Male   Female

Fig. 2.14 Center of gravity, male versus female.

2.10.1 Coxofemoral Joint

The coxofemoral joint consists of the acetabulum and the head of the femur (▶ Fig. 2.16). The skeletal pelvis not only supports and protects the abdominal and perineal viscera, but it is also a major component of the lower limbs. The skeletal pelvis serves to transfers its weight toand from the lower limbs, and the ground reaction forces are transmitted to the axial spine during locomotion. The rounded head of the femur articulates with the socket-shaped acetabulum of the hip, the coxofemoral joint. The head of the femur is spherical in nature and is covered with articular cartilage except for the indentation that is for the ligament of the femoral head. The acetabulum is formed by the fusion of the three bony components as discussed earlier

(▶ Fig. 2.17). A fibrocartilaginous acetabular labrum attaches to the acetabular rim effectively increasing the acetabular articulating surface area by nearly 10%.[2,4] The acetabular labrum bridges the acetabular notch resulting in more than half of the femoral head fitting within the acetabulum. The purpose of the acetabular labrum is to maintain integrity of the coxofemoral joint, fluid pressurization, and proprioception and to assist in dispersion of forces during weight-bearing activities.[2,4]

Tears to the acetabular labrum have been found to produces inguinal pain and are to be ruled out during the course of the evaluation when the history dictates that such a lesion may exist.[19,20]

> **Clinical Note**
>
> To test for labral integrity, the patient's hip is to be flexed to 90 degrees, maximally adducted, and internally rotated.

2.11 The Perineum[3,4]

The perineum, also designated the pelvic outlet, is the most caudal region of the axial body, and includes the skin of the inferior most glutei, medial most thighs, and external genitalia (▶ Fig. 2.18). The external genitalia of both the male and female should be understood as to their layout to to appreciate any unique characteristics that patients may present.

The skeletal limits of the perineum are as follows: the anterior limit is the pubic arch; the boundary outline continues laterally along the pubic and ischial rami to the ischial tuberosity and follows the STL to the tip of the coccyx bilaterally. The perineum is composed of two triangles, anteriorly the urogenital triangle, and posteriorly the anal triangle. Seen together they form a diamond shape. These two triangles do not lie on a single plane. An angle, when viewed from a lateral perspective, exists midway between the urogenital triangle anteriorly, and the anal triangle posteriorly.

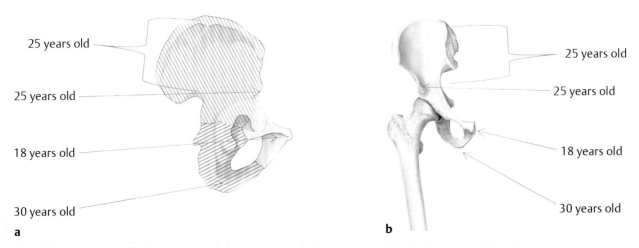

25 years old

25 years old

18 years old

30 years old

a

25 years old

25 years old

18 years old

30 years old

b

Fig. 2.15 a,b Epiphyses of the female pelvis. ([a] From Faller A, Schuenke M. The Human Body: An Introduction to Structure and Function, Thieme Publishers, Stuttgart: 2004. Used with permission.) ([b] From THIEME Atlas of Anatomy, General Anatomy and Musculoskeletal System, © Thieme 2005, illustration by Karl Wesker.)

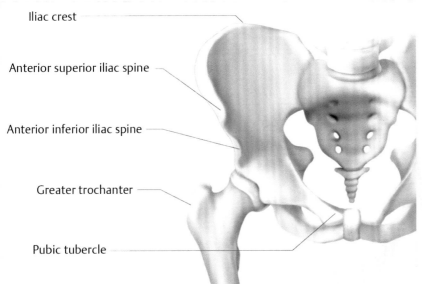

Iliac crest

Anterior superior iliac spine

Anterior inferior iliac spine

Greater trochanter

Pubic tubercle

Fig. 2.16 Coxofemoral joint. (From Reichert B. Palpation Techniques: Surface Anatomy for Physical Therapists, Thieme Publishers, Stuttgart: 2011. Used with permission.)

Learning Objectives

- The clinician will describe the three layers of the PFM.
- The clinician will apply the understanding of the three layers of the pelvic musculature during the course of the internal evaluation of the patient with pelvic pain.
- The clinician will identify the musculature of the pelvic floor based upon an understanding of its origin and insertion.

Confusion in terminology exists when discussing the contents of the urogenital triangle. Commonly referred to as the urogenital diaphragm, many argue the presence of an actual "diaphragm,"[21] stating that the muscles of the urogenital region do not form a diaphragmatic sheet, but extend through the visceral outlet into the lower reaches of the pelvic cavity; thus—in their opinion—there is no urogenital diaphragm as such.[22]

2.11.1 The Urogenital Triangle[2,4]

There is both a superficial and deep group of muscles in the urogenital triangle (▶ Fig. 2.19). The muscles of the deep perineal space include the deep transverse perineal muscle (transversus perinei profundus) and the sphincter urethrae muscle. The sphincter urethrae muscle surrounds the membraneous urethrae at the level of the deep perineal space and the neck of the bladder. In the male, central fibers continue into the prostate. The deep transverse perineal muscles take their origin from the ischial rami and cross laterally just anterior to the anus where they join the muscle of the other side. The perineal body, a focal attachment site of several muscles in the deep and superficial compartments, and a site of fusion of the inferior and superior fascial layers, is located in the midline between the anus and urogenital structures just superficial to the site of the intersection of fibers of the right and left transversus

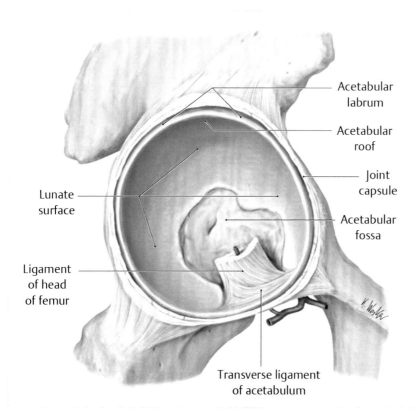

Fig. 2.17 Acetabulum. (From THIEME Atlas of Anatomy, General Anatomy and Musculoskeletal System, © Thieme 2005, illustration by Karl Wesker.)

Acetabular labrum

Acetabular roof

Joint capsule

Acetabular fossa

Lunate surface

Ligament of head of femur

Transverse ligament of acetabulum

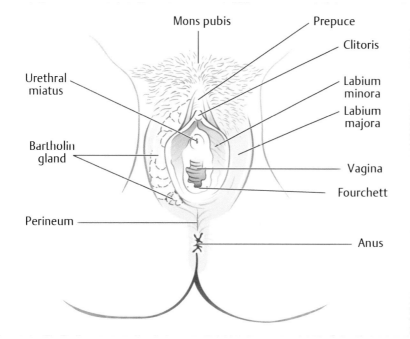

Fig. 2.18 Female external genitalia. (From Reece E, Barbieri R. Obstetrics and Gynecology: The Essentials of Clinical Care, Thieme Publishers, Stuttgart: 2010. Used with permission.)

Mons pubis

Prepuce

Clitoris

Labium minora

Labium majora

Urethral miatus

Bartholin gland

Vagina

Fourchett

Perineum

Anus

perinei profundus muscles. Muscle fibers and their fascia interlace to form the pyramidal-shaped perineal body and include all of the muscles of the deep and superficial groups as well as the smooth muscle of the internal anal sphincter.[2,4]

The muscles of the deep perineal space are covered inferiorly by the inferior fascia of the urogenital diaphragm, often referred to as the perineal membrane. The deep perineal space includes the deep perineal muscles, which are found between the superior fascia of the urogenital diaphragm and the inferior fascia of the urogenital diaphragm.

The muscles of the superficial perineal space include the superficial transverse perineal muscles, the paired bulbospongiosus muscles, and the paired ischiocavernosus muscles. The transversus perinei superficialis is a small strip of muscle that

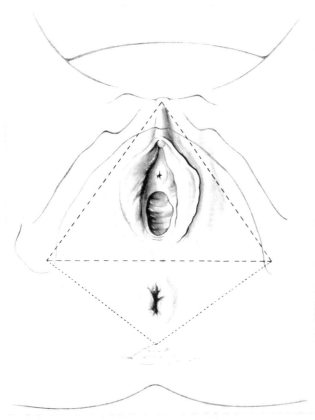

Fig. 2.19 Female urogenital triangle. (From Wallwiener D, Becker S, et al. Atlas of Gynecologic Surgery, Thieme Publishers, Stuttgart, 2014. Used with permission.)

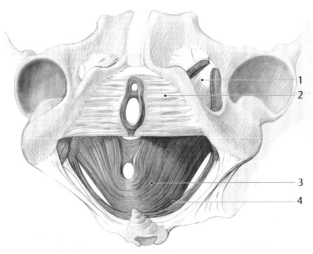

Fig. 2.20 The deep boundary between the vulvar region and the pelvis is shown. The illustration shows the urogenital diaphragm with the inferior fascia of the urogenital diaphragm (2) and the openings for the vagina and urethra. The adjacent muscle structures such as the bulbospongiosus ("vaginal sphincter") and the urethral sphincter are sketched. The different parts of the levator ani are shown posteriorly: iliococcygeus (lateral, 4) and pubococcygeus (medial, 3). The pubococcygeus passes superior to the urogenital diaphragm (and the superior fascia of the urogenital diaphragm that runs there) to its attachment in the pubic arch. The illustration does not show the gluteus maximus muscle to give a clear view of the complex of the sacrospinous ligament and sacrotuberous ligament (1). On the left, the obturator muscle has been divided in the obturator foramen so that the obturator fascia is visible. (From Wallwiener D, Becker S, et al. Atlas of Gynecologic Surgery, Thieme Publishers: Stuttgart, 2014. Used with permission.)

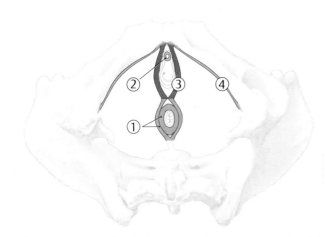

Fig. 2.21 Sphincters of perineum. (From THIEME Atlas of Anatomy, General Anatomy and Musculoskeletal System, © Thieme 2005, illustration by Karl Wesker.)

passes from each ischial tuberosity toward the midline where it inserts into the perineal body and fuses with fibers from the contralateral muscle. The bulbospongiosus is a midline muscle that consists of two parts joined by a median raphe (▶ Fig. 2.20).[2,4]

In the female, the bulbospongiosus muscle covers the superficial parts of the vestibular bulbs and greater vestibular glands and passes forward on either side of the vagina to attach to the body of the clitoris. The ischiocavernosus muscle originates from the ischial tuberosity and ramus but covers the crus of the clitoris.

The anal triangle contains the wedge-shaped ischiorectal fossa on either side of the anus, which houses two extensive fat pads that may be up to 10 cm thick.[23] The presence of these ischiorectal fat pads necessitates internal palpation and assessment as accurate palpation would be impossible through such a barrier. These fat pads are liquid at body temperature, which allows for easy distention of the rectum and anus during defecation. The pudendal nerves and internal pudendal artery and vein course through the ischiorectal fossa within a fascial compartment designated as Alcock's canal. Alcock's canal is a continuation of the obturator fascia and passes its contents forward along the inferior pubic rami.[2,4]

The external anal sphincter surrounds the lowest part of the anus and is bound to the overlying skin (▶ Fig. 2.21). The internal anal sphincter, although distinct from the anal triangle, is mentioned here to complete the anatomy of the anal sphincter as it functions with the external anal sphincter in fecal continence. Like all sphincters, the anal sphincters are closed in their relaxed state. The resting tone of these sphincters maintains closure of the anal canal lateral walls except during defecation and child birthing.[2,4]

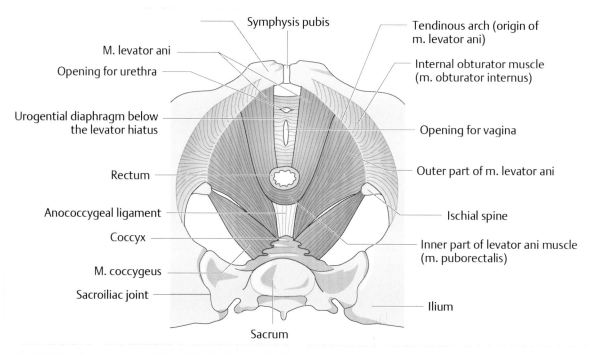

Symphysis pubis

M. levator ani

Opening for urethra

Urogential diaphragm below the levator hiatus

Rectum

Anococcygeal ligament

Coccyx

M. coccygeus

Sacroiliac joint

Sacrum

Tendinous arch (origin of m. levator ani)

Internal obturator muscle (m. obturator internus)

Opening for vagina

Outer part of m. levator ani

Ischial spine

Inner part of levator ani muscle (m. puborectalis)

Ilium

Fig. 2.22 Pelvic floor musculature. (From Faller A, Schuenke M. The Human Body: An Introduction to Structure and Function, Thieme Publishers, Stuttgart: 2004. Used with permission.)

2.12 Pelvic Musculature[2,4]

The PFM forms a hammock-like sling composed of the obturator internus muscle as the sidewalls, the two piriformis muscles as the posterior wall, with the pubic bones forming the anterior wall and the levator ani and coccygeal musculature forming the inferior aspect. A continuous sheath of parietal fascia envelopes the pelvic floor having originated from the transversalis fascia. The PFM plays a significant role in urethral function, urinary and fecal continence, support of the anus and lower third of the vagina and perineal body, visceral support, and sexual function.[2,4]

Learning Objectives

- The clinician will discuss the interaction of the PFM with the overall stability of the SIJ.
- The clinician will accurately appraise the evaluation findings as they relate to the integrity of the PFM.
- The clinician will label the PFM accurately.

The pelvic floor serves three distinct functions:
1. Plays supportive role in maintaining visceral alignment
2. Maintains fecal and urinary continence
3. Enhances sexual arousal and orgasm

Clinical Note

Knowing the origin and insertion of the pelvic musculature is of the upmost importance when it comes to accurately treating the patient with pelvic pain. The clinician is to demonstrate the ability to differentially palpate the musculature of the pelvic floor with this knowledge.

A collective sheet of striated musculature running from the coccyx posteriorly, and a tendinous arch of the obturator internus muscle laterally and from the inner surface of the superior rami of the pubic bones anteriorly form the inferior boundary of the pelvic cavity. The pelvic diaphragm can be divided into two components, the levator ani muscles anterior-laterally and the coccygeus muscles posteriorly (▶ Fig. 2.22). The levator ani muscle is further divided into the lateral iliococcygeus muscle and the anteromedial pubococcygeus muscle. The iliococcygeus muscles arise from that lateral inner surface of the coccyx and from a midline aponeurosis called the levator plate. The coccygeus muscles travel from the posterior portion of the cocyx and the lateral edges of the lower sacrum and terminate along the ischial spines. The pubococcygeus muscles arise from the medial inner surface of the coccyx and sacrum and the anterior sacrococcygeal ligament and the levator plate. Both muscles insert into the specialized tendinous arch of the levator ani muscle, which itself is suspended from the inner surface of the superior pubic ramus anteriorly and from the ischial spine posterolaterally. The tendinous arch of the levator ani muscle runs deep to the obturator internus muscle and inferior to the lateral region of the iliopectineal line of the pelvic brim and the obturator canal. The pubococcygeus muscle contains a subdivision medially that is designated the puborectalis muscle or puborectal sling (▶ Fig. 2.23). The puborectal sling originates from the posterior surface of the bodies of the pubic bones in a posterior fashion, wrapping around the anorectal hiatus and functions in bowel continence.

The musculature of the pelvic diaphragm is divided into three distinct layers (▶ Fig. 2.24), each roughly corresponding to the depth of a palpating knuckle. The first layer—also considered to be the urogenital triangle—consists of the superficial transverse perineal muscle and the ischiocavernosus and bulbocavernosus

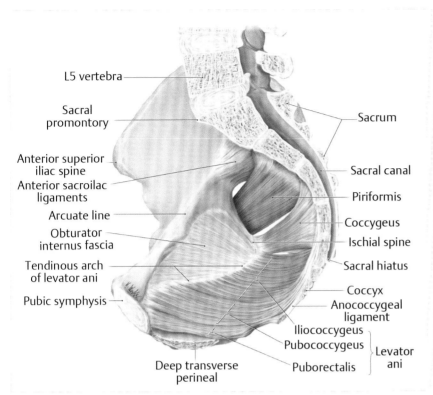

Fig. 2.23 Pelvic floor musculature, medial view. (From THIEME Atlas of Anatomy, General Anatomy and Musculoskeletal System, © Thieme 2005, illustration by Karl Wesker.)

L5 vertebra

Sacral promontory

Anterior superior iliac spine

Anterior sacroilac ligaments

Arcuate line

Obturator internus fascia

Tendinous arch of levator ani

Pubic symphysis

Deep transverse perineal

Sacrum

Sacral canal

Piriformis

Coccygeus

Ischial spine

Sacral hiatus

Coccyx

Anococcygeal ligament

Iliococcygeus

Pubococcygeus

Puborectalis

Levator ani

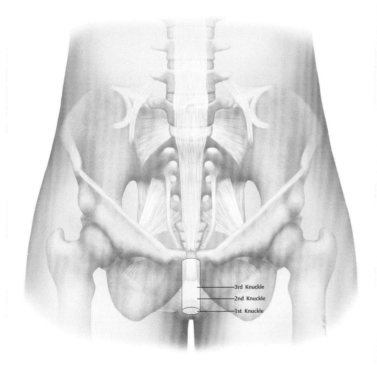

Fig. 2.24 a,b Three layers of pelvic musculature palpation.

3rd Knuckle
2nd Knuckle
1st Knuckle

Fig. 2.24 (*Continued*)

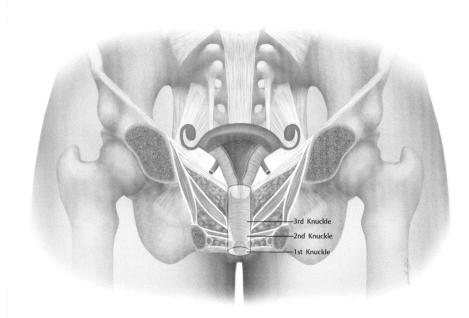

3rd Knuckle
2nd Knuckle
1st Knuckle

musculature. Surrounding structures include the urethra, lower vagina, vulva, mons pubis, labia majora and minora, clitoris, vestibular bulb, and Bartholin's glands. The second layer, also a component of the urogenital diaphragm, consists of the sphincter urethrae, deep transverse perineal muscle, and compressor urethrae. Local structures include the Bartholin's glands, urethra, perineal membrane, and vagina. The third layer, also referred to as the pelvic diaphragm, consists of the levator ani (pubococcygeus, puborectalis, and iliococcygeus), obturator internus, and ischiococcygeus/coccygeus. Local structures include the tendionous arch of the levator ani musculature, obturator fascia, and the sacrotuberous and sacrospinous ligaments (SSLs).

The female and male pelvic diaphragms are similar in construct, both demonstrating a large anterior hiatus; the differences are that the female pelvic diaphragm contains the deep dorsal veins of the clitoris, the urethra, and the vagina, whereas in males the pelvic diaphragm contains the deep dorsal veins of the penis and the urethra.

Embryological studies confirm that the puborectalis muscle is a portion of the levator ani. The primordium, an organ or tissue in its earliest recognizable stage of development, makes no differentiation between the ilio- and pubococcygeus muscles.[24] According to Barber et al, the levator ani is not innervated by the pudendal nerve, but the study evaluated female subjects only. Innervation was found to occur directly from roots that travel along the superior surface of the pelvic floor. This was confirmed in vivo with nerve conduction studies in humans, and further confirmed with dissection.[25] This contradicts other sources that discuss a "dual" innervation by branches from the pudendal nerve and direct branches S3–5.

Several structures pass through the pelvic diaphragm including the rectum, the urethra, and the vagina. The most posterior of these pelvic effluents is the rectum, which is surrounded by bands of muscle called the puborectalis muscle. These muscles originate on either side of the posterior aspect of the body of the pubis and pass posteriorly to join muscle fibers on the con-tralateral side behind the rectum. The puborectalis joins the external anal sphincter and forms a sling around the rectum, producing a flexure at the anal-rectal junction.

The puborectalis muscle is barely distinct from the pubococcygeus muscle at the posterior side of the pubic bodies where both muscles originate. However, the pubococcygeus passes posteriorly in a plane superior to that traversed by the puborectalis and inserts on the anterior surface of the coccyx. Certain portions of the pubococcygeus muscle are assigned names that specify their insertion into other structures as the whole muscle passes posteriorly toward the coccyx. These include the fibers that insert into the sphincter urethrae (in the male into the prostate, into the vagina in females, and into the perineal body and the rectum in both males and females).

The iliococcygeus muscle is that part of the levator ani that takes its origin from the band of tissue on the internal fascia of the obturator internus muscle known as the arcus tendinous and from the ischial spine. This muscle extends posteromedially to insert on the final segments of the coccyx.

The coccygeus muscle, which together with the levator ani compose the pelvic diaphragm, lies on the anterior surface of the SSL. Its attachments are the ischial spine laterally and the coccyx posteriorly, and it is innervated by sacral nerves 3 and 4.[2,4]

A thorough understanding of the interrelationship of the external musculature and its effect on the pelvis and pelvic floor is paramount in the clinician's evaluation of patients with pelvic pain. It is common for the suffering patient to have developed compensatory restrictions throughout the coxofemoral joint and its musculature.[4]

Both the piriformis and obturator internus serve dual functions: locomotion and maintaining homeostasis of the pelvic floor. Due to their origin along the inner surface of the pelvic bones, and especially with the obturator internus as an origin of the lateral aspect of the pelvic floor, tension through one or both will have an immediate effect on the length tension of the pelvic floor.[4]

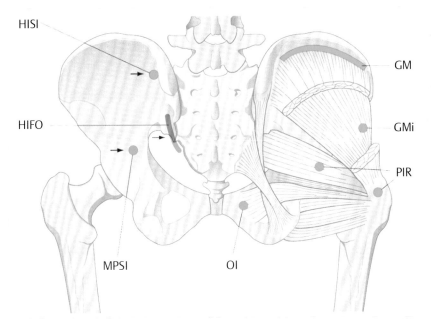

HISI

HIFO

MPSI

OI

GM

GMi

PIR

Fig. 2.25 Tender points in the posterior pelvis and hip. Note: the arrows point in the direction of palpation. GM: gluteus medius; GMI: gluteus minimus; HIFO: high ilium with flare-out; HISI: high ilium sacroiliac; MPSI: midpole sacroiliac; OI: obturator internus; PIR: piriformis. (From Carriere B, Feldt CM. The Pelvic Floor, Thieme Publishers, Stuttgart: 2006. Used with permission.)

The obturator internus originates along the inner edges of the obturator internus foramina, exiting through the lesser sciatic foramina and inserting on the greater trochanter of the femur (▶ Fig. 2.25). The piriformis originates along the inner surface of the lower portion of the sacral ala, exiting the pelvis through the greater sciatic foramina, with its insertion being above that of the obturator internus muscle on the greater trochanter. All somatic innervation is provided by branches of the lumbosacral plexus.[4]

The piriformis muscle is a strong lateral rotator of the thigh. It is a large muscle that covers the lateral portions of sacral vertebrae 2, 3, and 4 just lateral to the pelvic foramina of each respective vertebra. Originating on the pelvic surface of the sacrum, the piriformis muscle leaves the pelvis through the greater sciatic foramen and attaches to the medial side of the most superior point of the greater trochanter of the femur. The piriformis is innervated by sacral nerves 1 and 2 through small branches of the sacral plexus.[4]

The obturator internus muscle originates within the pelvis on the obturator membrane, and on portions of the ischium and ilium, lateral to the obturator foramen. Though broad in origin, the muscle merges to a narrow tendon that passes through the lesser sciatic foramen and rides over the ischial body superior to the ischial tuberosity attaching on the medial aspect of the greater trochanter of the femur. The gemelli muscles flank the tendon of the obturator internus muscle as they pass from their origin on the posterior aspect of the ischial body (superior gemellus from the ischial spine, inferior gemellus from the ischial tuberosity) and insert into the tendon of the obturator internus muscle; both gemelli muscles are lateral rotators. The obturator internus originates from the obturator membrane and runs primarily laterally, turning sharply lateral over the ischium, making a nearly 90-degree turn. The obturator internus muscle is innervated by sacral nerves 1 and 2 through small branches of the sacral plexus. A major part of the pelvic diaphragm attaches to the fascia of the obturator internus.[4]

Clinical Note

The obturator internus refers pain to the inguinal region and lateral gluteal regions.

The obturator externus muscle takes its origin from the external or anterior surface of the obturator membrane and from the bone that surrounds the obturator foramen. As per the obturator internus, the obturator externus converges to a slim tendon over the ischium and passes superiorly behind the femoral neck to insert on the trochanteric fossa of the femur. The obturator externus muscle is primarily a lateral rotator of the thigh and is innervated by the obturator nerve.[4]

2.13 Pelvic Ligaments[4]

The pelvis and pelvic ring are supported by a series of ligaments, some of which serve a secondary function as attachment sites for the local musculature. From the anterior perspective (▶ Fig. 2.26), there is a pair of inguinal ligaments that run from the anterior superior iliac spine (ASIS) to the ipsilateral pubic tubercle. These ligaments form the inferior border of the aponeurosis of the internal oblique muscle and serve as the floor of the inguinal canal.

From a posterior perspective (▶ Fig. 2.27) there is a pair of sacroiliac ligaments and an iliolumbar ligament, which assist in the stabilization of the SIJ. Covering the anterior and posterior sacroiliac joints are the anterior and posterior sacroiliac ligaments, respectively.

The STL and the SSL cross the sacral inlet from the lateral surface of the sacrum to the more laterally placed ischial tuberosity and ischial spine, respectively. These ligaments are extremely strong and will often feel ossified during palpation making a distinction between osseous structures and ligament difficult. The STL has extensive connections with the gluteus maximus,

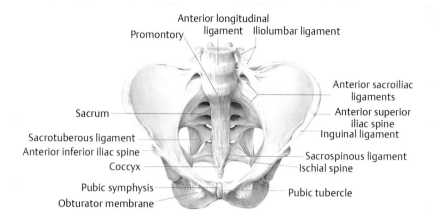

Anterior longitudinal
ligament   Iliolumbar ligament
Promontory

Sacrum

Sacrotuberous ligament
Anterior inferior iliac spine
Coccyx
Pubic symphysis
Obturator membrane

Anterior sacroiliac
ligaments
Anterior superior
iliac spine
Inguinal ligament

Sacrospinous ligament
Ischial spine

Pubic tubercle

Fig. 2.26 Anterior pelvic ligaments. (From THIEME Atlas of Anatomy, General Anatomy and Musculoskeletal System, © Thieme 2005, illustration by Karl Wesker.)

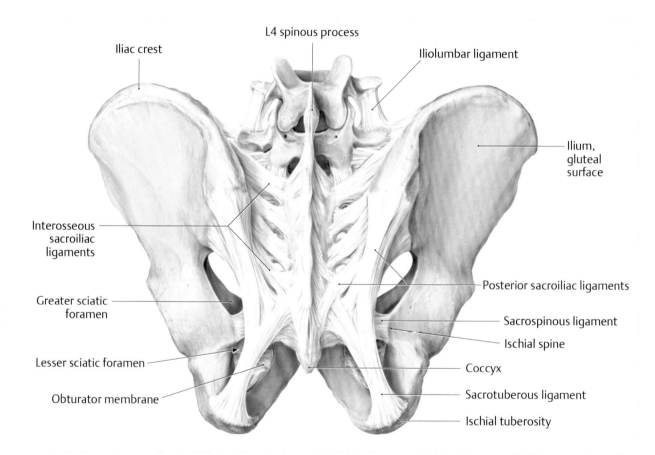

Iliac crest

L4 spinous process

Iliolumbar ligament

Ilium,
gluteal
surface

Interosseous
sacroiliac
ligaments

Greater sciatic
foramen

Lesser sciatic foramen

Obturator membrane

Posterior sacroiliac ligaments

Sacrospinous ligament

Ischial spine

Coccyx

Sacrotuberous ligament

Ischial tuberosity

Fig. 2.27 Posterior pelvic ligaments. (From THIEME Atlas of Anatomy, General Anatomy and Musculoskeletal System, © Thieme 2005, illustration by Karl Wesker.)

the long head of the biceps femoris, the iliococcygeus muscle, and the SSL. Nutation (anterior rotation of ilium relative to the sacrum) will result in tension of the STL, whereas counternutation will slacken it. Conversely, the SSL will restrict nutation (posterior rotation of the ilium relative to the sacrum). The STL and SSL cross when viewed posteriorly, with the STL being more posterior-lateral. The STL is longer than the SSL. The space between the dorsal sacroiliac ligament and the interosseous

sacroiliac ligament is large enough to accommodate the dorsal rami of sacral nerves and blood vessels that pass through.

Learning Objectives

- The clinician will recall the ligaments of the pelvic ring.
- The clinician will identify the location of the ligaments of the pelvic ring on a skeletal model.

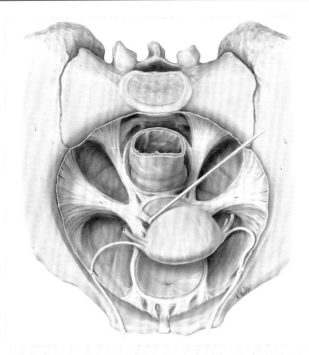

Fig. 2.28 Visceral ligaments. (From Atlas of Anatomy, © Thieme 2008–2012, illustration by Karl Wesker.)

The long posterior sacroiliac ligament arises from the intermediate sacral crest with the lower part arising from the lateral crest.[26] The superficial fibers run almost vertically from the third and fourth sacral transverse tubercles to the posterior superior iliac spine and internal end of the iliac crest and functions as a means of limiting counternutation. The iliolumbar ligament originates from the transverse process of L4 and L5 and anchors the transverse process of L5 to the iliac crest and sacrum. Minor deformities due to a disk lesion can lead to significant pain. The SSL closes off the bony component of the greater sciatic notch creating the greater sciatic foramen, whereas the STL forms the inferomedial border of the greater sciatic foramen. The SSL forms the superior border of the lesser sciatic foramen.

The STL is found between the posterior iliac spines, the lower part of the sacrum, and the upper coccyx. The fibers run obliquely down and lateral inserting at the medial margin of the ischial tuberosity. The gluteus maximus, thoracolumbar fascia, multifidus muscle, and long head biceps femoris have ligamentous origins. Functionally, it limits nutation. The anterior sacroiliac ligament provides anterior stability to the SIJ and is readily palpated and treated via internal palpation techniques that are described in Chapter 5. This ligament has been found to be a common cause of a patient's persistent lower back pain and SIJ dysfunction.

Support to the vagina and the uterus is created by the subserous fascia within the pelvic floor that thickens to form the ligaments of the uterus (anterior vesicouterine ligaments, posterior uterosacral ligaments, and lateral transverse cervical ligaments, Mackenrodt's ligament, cardinal ligaments) (▶ Fig. 2.28).[2,4] The vesicouterine ligaments are thickened bands of subserous fascia that course from the lateral walls of the base of the uterus to the base of the bladder. The uterosacral ligaments are thickened bands of the subserous fascia and muscle fibers that course from the base of the uterus to the sacrum and are enclosed within the lateral uterosacral folds that form the lateral borders of the pararectal fossae. The transverse cervical ligaments are thickened bands of subserous fascia that course within the inferior roots of the broad ligaments and connect the lateral walls of the base of the uterus to the pelvis in the regions of the SIJs at the medial surfaces of the psoas muscles. The uterine artery and vein, which provide vasculature to the uterus, originate as the internal iliac artery and vein. The uterus is further supported by the fibers of the levator ani muscle, the urogenital diaphragm, and the transverse perineal muscles and perineal body.

The urethra is found at the base of the bladder and drains the urine to the outside of the body. In males the urethra has three parts: prostatic urethra, membranous urethra, and penile urethra. In females the urethra has only the membranous urethra, which is about as long as the prostatic and membranous urethras in males combined. The base of the bladder is supported by subserous fascia.[2,4] These are thickened bands on either side of the bladder that in the male are the puboprostatic ligament and in the female the pubovesical ligament; they are commonly referred to as "false ligaments," inclusive of the medial umbilical ligament, which is covered by the median umbilical fold.

2.14 Neurology[2,3,4,27,28]

Knowledge of the origin and function of the nervous system helps the clinician understand the origin of the patient's pain and how the pain is referred to a location other than its source.[1,2,3,4]

Learning Objectives

- The clinician will recall the various neurological structures that represent the patient with pelvic pain, and the viscera.
- The clinician will compare the patient's presentation with his or her knowledge of neurological anatomy.
- The clinician will explain the patient's pain presentation as it relates to the neuroanatomy.

The CNS consists primarily of the brain and spinal cord. Together they integrate and control the body with relationship to the environment and activity. This is accomplished through several columns and tracks that carry specific information regarding that status of their host including muscle, viscous, joint, and so forth.

The dorsal column carries information regarding graphesthesia, two-point discrimination, positional sense, and visceral pain; a limited midline myelotomy has been shown to be effective in the reduction of intractable pelvic cancer pain in humans (▶ Fig. 2.29).[27,28] The dorsal column demonstrates a somatotopic arrangement as it relates to the viscera, responding to both mechanical and chemical irritation.[29,30] Conversely, excruciating pain in the sacral region and perineum is experienced when the dorsal column or medial aspect of the nucleus gracilis is probed mechanically. Nociceptive activity from uterine and vaginal distension is found within the dorsal column nuclei, and can be triggered by unmyelinated primary afferent fibers that ascend the dorsal column directly to the dorsal column nuclei or they may be mediated through the postsynaptic

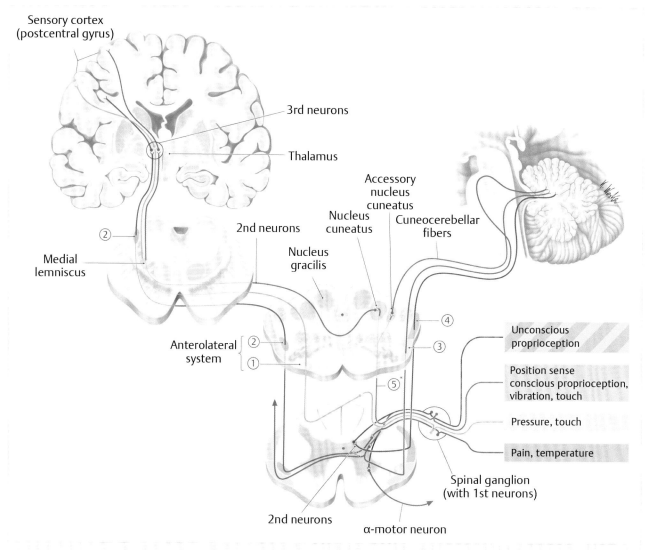

Sensory cortex
(postcentral gyrus)

3rd neurons

Thalamus

Accessory
nucleus
cuneatus

Nucleus
cuneatus

Cuneocerebellar
fibers

2nd neurons

②

Medial
lemniscus

Nucleus
gracilis

Anterolateral
system

②
①

④

③

⑤*

Unconscious
proprioception

Position sense
conscious proprioception,
vibration, touch

Pressure, touch

Pain, temperature

Spinal ganglion
(with 1st neurons)

2nd neurons

α-motor neuron

Fig. 2.29 Dorsal column. (From Atlas of Anatomy, © Thieme 2008–2012, illustration by Karl Wesker.)

dorsal column pathway. The dorsal column pathway originates from cells in lamina III and lamina X. In contrast to the spinothalamic tract cells, the postsynaptic dorsal column cells are innervated by serotonin reactive fibers.

Stimulation of the Meissner's corpuscles, Merkel cells, Ruffini endings, and Pacinian corpuscles located in the skin initiate an action potential that travels through the dorsal root ganglion and enters the dorsal column at the respective level, based on the dermatome stimulated. Nociceptive projection neurons in the spinal cord transmit information to the brain stem, diencephalon (inclusive of the thalamus, periaqueductal gray, parabrachial region, and bulbar reticular formation) and limbic structures in the hypothalamus, amygdaloidal nucleus, and septal nucleus.

Cell bodies of the spinal afferent primary neurons, such as the DRG, synapse at the level of the dorsal column of the spinal cord. There they travel via dorsal columns and the medial and lateral spinothalamic tracts. The "lateral system" consists of the lateral spinothalamic tract and its higher projections and processes sensory discriminative aspects of pain: location and intensity.

Clinical Note

Schmorl's nodes: Vertebral endplate fractures
- Occur most frequently between T8 and L2
- Initially felt as a "deep ache"; decrease with time
- May present themselves ten or more years later
- May be a contributing factor to Pelvic pain and dysfunction
- Embryogenetic origin of multiple visceral structures arise between T8-L2

The hypogastric nerves are the preganglionic sympathetic fibers and visceral afferent fibers from the thoracic, lumbar and sacral splanchnic nerves (▶ Fig. 2.30). Parasympathetic fibers from the pelvic splanchnic nerves connect the superior and inferior hypogastric plexuses. The superior hypogastric plexus originates at the level of T10 to L2, providing the viscous of the pelvis with preganglionic sympathetic fibers. The superior hypogastric plexus (presacral nerve) contains sympathetic fibers that supply the ureteral, ovarian, common iliac and

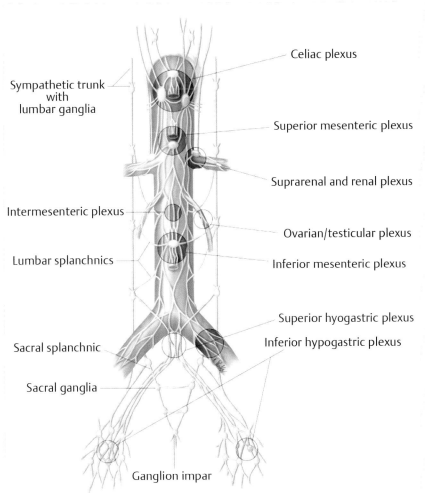

Celiac plexus

Sympathetic trunk
with
lumbar ganglia

Superior mesenteric plexus

Suprarenal and renal plexus

Intermesenteric plexus

Ovarian/testicular plexus

Lumbar splanchnics

Inferior mesenteric plexus

Superior hyogastric plexus

Inferior hypogastric plexus

Sacral splanchnic

Sacral ganglia

Ganglion impar

Fig. 2.30 Thoracolumbosacral plexus. (From Atlas of Anatomy, © Thieme 2008–2012, illustration by Karl Wesker.)

inferior hypogastric plexuses, while the inferior hypogastric plexus gives rise to three additional plexuses: the rectal plexus that travels to the rectum; the uterovaginal plexus that innervates the uterus, cervix, and vagina; and the vesicle plexus that innervates the bladder and vesicle blood vessels. This plexus contains both sympathetic and parasympathetic ganglia. Additionally, many afferent fibers from the bladder, uterus, and lower rectum pass through this region as they continue on to their respective dorsal root ganglia. Pain from the uterus is often referred to neuronal distributions supplied by the sacral nerves and T12 causing pain that is referred to the lower back, pubic, inguinal or anterior thigh areas.[31]

Nerves from the inferior hypogastric plexus and the uterovaginal plexus innervate the clitoris, vagina and vestibular glands and are generally parasympathetic fibers that are primarily responsible for vasodilation (▶ Fig. 2.31). The ovary has its own visceral innervation; the parasympathetic supply comes from the vagus nerve and the sympathetic supply from the pre-aortic plexus. The ovaries receive innervation from the ovarian plexus, a network of visceral nerves from T10 and T11; refers pain to T10 and T11 dermatomes. In general, pain originating from any of the pelvic organs can refer to the low anterior abdominal wall, low back, inguinal, and anterior thigh regions. Three nociceptive pathways from the pelvis convey their information through the inferior hypogastric plexus and is considered to be

a 'major autonomic relay center of the pelvis', integrating both sympathetic and parasympathetic output.[31]

The vagus nerve, cranial nerve X, innervates the entire gastrointestinal tract with exception of the distal third of the colon. The cell bodies of the vagal afferent primary neurons lie in the ganglion nodosum and synapse with second order neurons in the nucleus tractus solitarii (NTS), which is the main sensory nucleus of the vagus nerve. The majority of information is conveyed to the parabrachial nucleus (PBN) in the pons, where fibers ascend to visceral sensory cortical areas via the ventral posterior medial nucleus of the thalamus, and to regions of the brain that regulate arousal and emotions: hypothalamus, amygdale and antero- cingulate cortex. Sensory information is further modulated and processed with information regarding long-term memory, emotional valence of intero- and exteroceptive stimuli.

The peripheral nervous system provides a means to which the appendicular structures communicate with the CNS through afferent nerves, those that bring information toward the CNS, and efferent division of nerves, those that conduct information from the CNS to their respective effector cells; muscles and glands (▶ Fig. 2.32). The efferent division is further broken down into the somatic nervous system and the autonomic nervous system. The somatic nervous system innervates the skin, joints and muscles and is responsible for conducting

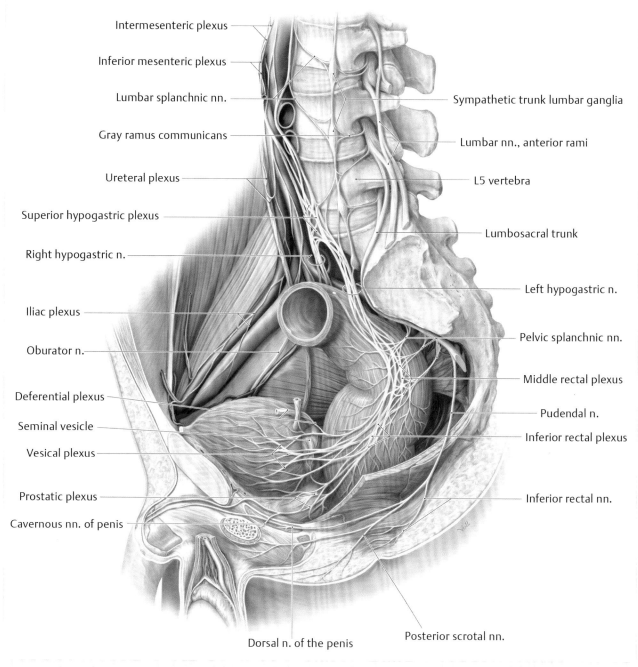

Intermesenteric plexus

Inferior mesenteric plexus

Lumbar splanchnic nn.

Gray ramus communicans

Ureteral plexus

Superior hypogastric plexus

Right hypogastric n.

Iliac plexus

Oburator n.

Deferential plexus

Seminal vesicle

Vesical plexus

Prostatic plexus

Cavernous nn. of penis

Dorsal n. of the penis

Sympathetic trunk lumbar ganglia

Lumbar nn., anterior rami

L5 vertebra

Lumbosacral trunk

Left hypogastric n.

Pelvic splanchnic nn.

Middle rectal plexus

Pudendal n.

Inferior rectal plexus

Inferior rectal nn.

Posterior scrotal nn.

Fig. 2.31 Pelvic innervation. (From Atlas of Anatomy, © Thieme 2008–2012, illustration by Markus Voll.)

information involving voluntary motor control. The autonomic nervous system (ANS) is responsible for controlling those actions that are involuntary in nature, including cardiac muscle function, smooth muscle function and glandular activity (▶ Fig. 2.33). The ANS is further subdivided into the sympathetic division and the parasympathetic division.

The sympathetic nervous system is primary responsible for mobilizing the body's resources under stressful situations; the flight-or-fight response. Also known as the thoracolumbar system,[3,4] the sympathetic nervous system originates from the intermediolateraly gray columns of T1-L2 regions of the spinal cord and reduces digestive secretions, increases heart rate and

contracts blood vessels. The sympathetic axons exit the spinal foramen through a small branch known as the white ramus communicans which connects to a series of ganglia, which in turn forms a chain of ganglia, one ganglia corresponding to each nerve root level. The glands and smooth muscle cells of the head, neck, heart, trachea, bronchi, and viscera of the abdomino-pelvic cavity and perineum are provided with sympathetic innervation by specialized visceral nerves that emanate from these chain ganglia and are given specific names for each component.

Splanchnic nerves which innervate the abdominal, pelvic and perineal viscera through prevertebral ganglia are located within

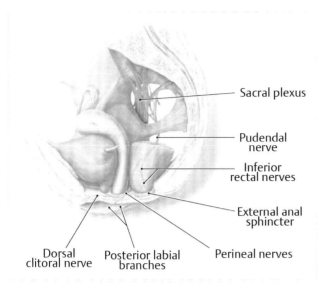

Fig. 2.32 Pelvic peripheral nerves. (From THIEME Atlas of Anatomy, General Anatomy and Musculoskeletal System, © Thieme 2005, illustration by Karl Wesker.)

the target viscous. Many names are used to describe these pre-aortic ganglia: celiac, superior mesenteric, aortic renal and inferior mesenteric ganglia. These preaortic ganglia are innervated by preganglionic fibers from special sympathetic splanchnic nerves that exit directly from chain ganglia at the thoracic and lumbar levels, descending along the vertebral column, piercing the diaphragm as they enter into the abdominal cavity. The greater *splanchnic nerve, a division of the splanchnic nerve,* is located at T4/5 to T9 and enters the abdominal cavity through a specialized foramen of the diaphragm and innervates peripheral sympathetic neurons within the celiac ganglia. These fibers modulate the enteric nervous system of the foregut- region from mouth to duodenum while also providing sympathetic innervations to the adrenal medulla. The lesser splanchnic nerve is composed of preganglionic fibers arising from T11 and/ or T12 and innervate peripheral sympathetic neurons within the aortic renal ganglia which then gives off postganglionic fibers that innervate the kidneys and suprarenal glands as they accompany the arteries to these organs. The lesser splanchnic modulates the activity of the enteric nervous system of the midgut- duodenum to approximately two-thirds through the transverse colon. The lumbar splanchnic nerve arises from L1 and 2, sometimes 3, and innervates the peripheral sympathetic neurons within the inferior mesenteric ganglia. Fibers from the ganglia follow branches of the inferior mesenteric artery to innervate the remaining one-third of the transverse colon, descending and sigmoid colon, the rectum and the pelvic viscera. The pelvic splanchnic nerves arise from S2–4 and provide innervation to the hindgut. The pelvic splanchnic nerves travel to their corresponding hypogastric plexus, which is located bilaterally on the walls of the rectum. They regulate the emptying of the bladder and rectum, in addition to carrying information regarding sexual arousal from the clitoris and penis alike.[3,4]

The parasympathetic nervous system is responsible for those actions that oppose physiological effects of the sympathetic nervous system: stimulates digestive secretions, slows the heart, constricts the pupils, dilates blood vessels, increases intestinal and glandular activity, and relaxes sphincter contractions. The parasympathetic nervous system originates in the brain stem and lower part of the spinal cord; central neurons are located in the brainstem in association with cranial nerves III, VII, IX, and X and the gray matter of the spinal cord levels S2–4 and is accepted as the true 'cranio-sacral system'. Unlike the sympathetic nervous system with its chain like organization of ganglia along the vertebral column, the parasympathetic nervous ganglia are embedded within the confines of the target tissue. Normal micturition, defecation and sexual function are under parasympathetic control arising from S2–4. The parasympathetic nervous system in the pelvis is carried by the pelvic splanchnic nerves that arise from the sacral spinal cord.[3,4]

Innervation to the anterior and lateral abdominal wall, down to the level of the mons pubis, originates from the 7th to 11th intercostal nerves (T7-T11), the subcostal nerve (T12) and the iliohypogastric and ilioinguinal nerves from the L1 branch of the lumbar plexus (▶ Fig. 2.34). Branches from T7 extend throughout the anterior wall to the level of the xiphoid process, T10 extends and includes the umbilicus and nerves from L1 innervate the level of the mons pubis. Posteriorly, branches from T10 and T11 innervate the lower lumbar region and upper portion of the sacrum; lateral cutaneous branches from the subcostal and iliohypogastric nerves supply the gluteal region.[32]

Clinical Note

Remember the concepts of peripheral sensitization when evaluating the patient with pelvic pains. One dermatome can spread to another, often requiring a treatment to be applied to a spinal segment that otherwise may not refer to the patient's reported pain local.

Mononeuropathies are the most common variant of chronic abdomino-pelvic pain.[13] The peripheral nerve may be injured by mechanical pressure or ischemia as they pass through ligamentous or fascial bands as a result of faulty body mechanics, and/or local injury (sports, motor vehicle accident, trauma, surgical). Any of the branches of the peripheral nervous system can become entrapped; however, the most common are the iliohypogastric and ilioinguinal nerves.[3,4]

The lumbar plexus, L1 to L4, provides somatic innervation to the lower abdominal wall and thighs. Branches of the lumbarsacral plexus include the iliohypogastric and ilioinguinal nerves (L1), the genitocrural nerve (L1–2) and the obturator nerve (L2–4). The iliohypogastric nerve innervates the skin above the pubic bone inclusive of the mons pubis and the adjacent transverse abdominis and internal oblique musculature. Traveling just caudal to the iliohypogastric nerve, the ilioinguinal nerve innervates the mons pubis and the anterior aspect of the labia majora and medial thigh. The lateral femoral cutaneous nerve (L2–3) carries sensory information from the lateral gluteal muscles to the anterolateral thigh to the knee, and to the parietal peritoneum of the iliac fossa. Originating from T11 to L1, this nerve emerges from the upper, lateral aspect of the psoas major and runs parallel to the 12 fth thoracic nerve and anterior to the quadratus lumborum, where, at the crest of the ilium it divides into the iliac and hypogastric nerves, supplying the hypogastric and suprapubic skin. Muscular branches innervate

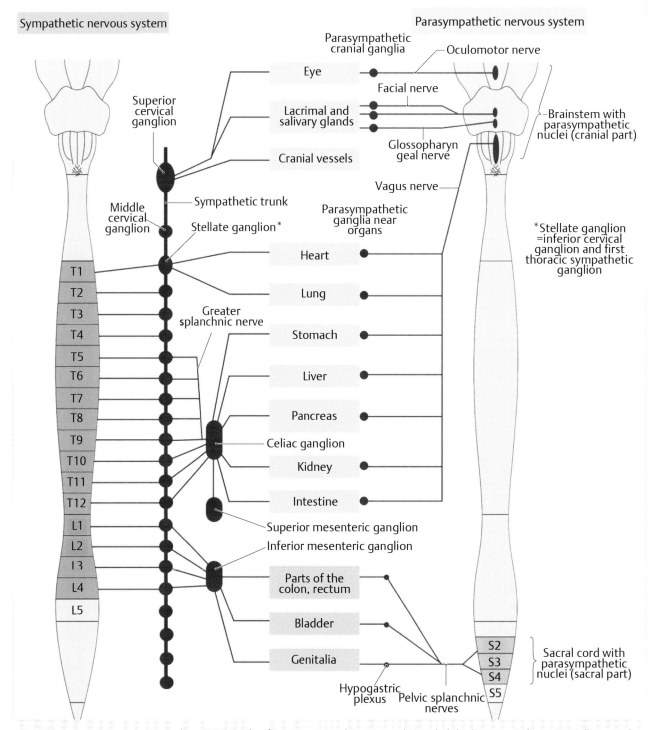

Fig. 2.33 Autonomic nervous system. (From THIEME Atlas of Anatomy, General Anatomy and Musculoskeletal System, © Thieme 2005, illustration by Markus Voll.)

the transversalis, internal, and external oblique muscles. Arising from the T12 to L1 nerve roots this nerve runs parallel of the iliohypgastric to the inguinal canal, where it emerges through the external abdominal ring or the external pillar of the ring.[3,4]

Originating from L1–2, the genitofemoral nerve consists primarily of sensory fibers and travels within the fascial lining of the abdominal cavity, piercing the psoas muscle and fascia at the level of L3–4, dividing into the terminal genital and femoral branches distal to the inguinal ligament. The genital branch (primarily L1) traverses the inguinal canal with the round ligament reaching the labia majora. The femoral branch (primarily L2) provides sensation to the labia major, inguinal region, and upper medial thigh.

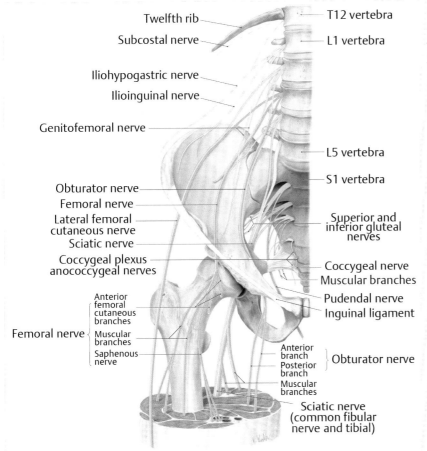

Twelfth rib

Subcostal nerve

Iliohypogastric nerve

Ilioinguinal nerve

Genitofemoral nerve

Obturator nerve

Femoral nerve

Lateral femoral cutaneous nerve

Sciatic nerve

Coccygeal plexus anococcygeal nerves

Anterior femoral cutaneous branches

Femoral nerve { Muscular branches

Saphenous nerve

T12 vertebra

L1 vertebra

L5 vertebra

S1 vertebra

Superior and inferior gluteal nerves

Coccygeal nerve

Muscular branches

Pudendal nerve

Inguinal ligament

Anterior branch
Posterior branch } Obturator nerve

Muscular branches

Sciatic nerve (common fibular nerve and tibial)

Fig. 2.34 Innervation of anterior and lateral abdomen and thigh. (From THIEME Atlas of Anatomy, General Anatomy and Musculoskeletal System, © Thieme 2005, illustration by Karl Wesker.)

Arising from the fibers of L2–3, the lateral femoral cutaneous nerve runs downward over the iliacus muscle, through the iliac fossa, under the iliac fascia, and it descends into the tensor fascia lata and further divides into an anterior and posterior terminal branch innervating the anterolateral and posterior thigh.

Originating from L2–4 with infrequent contributions from L1 and L5, the roots unite within the psoas major, passing downward and finally outward to anterolateral of the pelvis above the obturator vessels, and finally dividing into its terminal anterior and posterior braches and a branch to the obturator externus. The obturator nerve (L2–4) innervates the adductor musculature and the cutaneous region of the medial aspect of the thigh.

The femoral nerve (L1–4) is the largest branch of the lumbar plexus, innervating the quadriceps femoris, Sartorius, and pectineus muscles. Cutaneous branches innervate the medial and anterior thigh, groin, hip, and knee joints.[3,4,13]

The genitocrural nerve (L1–2) provides cutaneous innervations to the anterior thigh and mons pubis.

The sacral plexus (L4-S4) innervates the levator ani, obturator internus, coccygeus, piriformis, and gemellus and quadrates femoris musculature. The superior/inferior gluteal nerves, pudendal nerve, posterior femoral cutaneous nerve, and the sciatic nerve are all derived from the sacral plexus. The sciatic nerve (L4-S3) innervates the hamstring musculature and

gastrocnemius muscle with branches (peroneal) that provide cutaneous innervation to the lateral aspect of the lower leg.

Arising from the S2–4 nerve roots, the pudendal nerve passes between the piriformis muscle and cocygeus leaving the pelvis through the greater sciatic foramen, under the sciatic nerve. It then passes forward with the internal pudendal artery and nerve to cross the base of the lesser SSL and enters the fascial tunnel known as Alcock's canal in the obturator fascia on the inferior-medial most aspect of the ischial tuberosity. It then divides into its terminal branches: perineal nerve and dorsal clitoral nerve. Roots of the pudendal nerve leave the pelvic foramen of sacral vertebrae 2, 3, and 4 on the pelvic surface and join to form the nerve proper. Once formed, the nerve leaves the pelvis via the greater sciatic foramen and enters the perineum using the lesser sciatic foramen, and then finds its way to its target organs without penetrating the pelvic diaphragm. The pudendal nerve provides sensation to the external genitalia, containing both somatic efferent and afferent fibers, and sympathetic and parasympathetic efferents and visceral afferents.

The anococcygeal nerve provides sensation to the perineum between the coccyx and the anus; whereas the cutaneous branch of the inferior rectal nerve gives rise to sensation to the anus, the perineal branch of the posterior femoral cutaneous nerves provides innervation to the lateral labia majora and branches of the perineal nerve innervate the medial labia (▶ Fig. 2.35; ▶ Table 2.2).

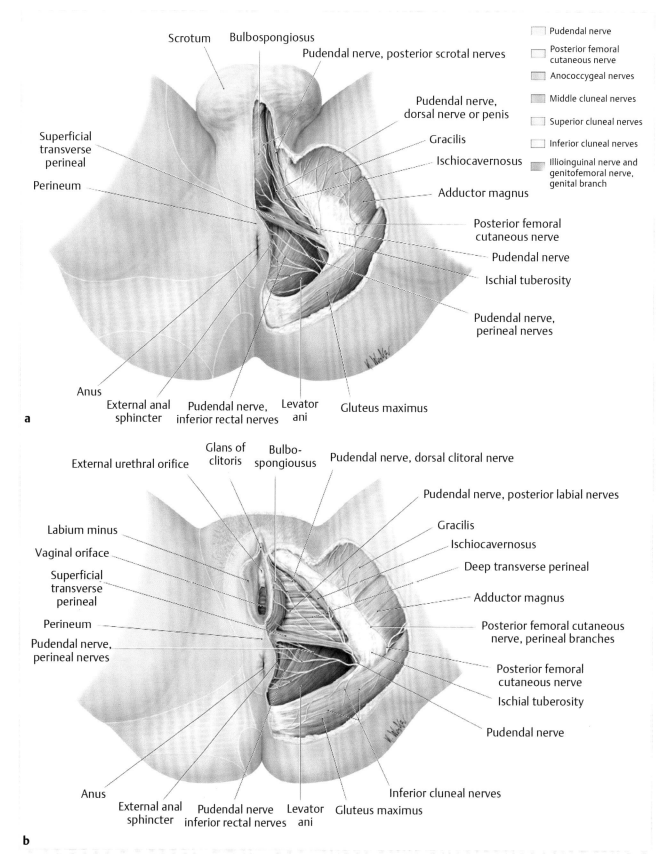

Fig. 2.35 a,b Summary of somatic and cutaneous innervation.[82] (From THIEME Atlas of Anatomy, General Anatomy and Musculoskeletal System, © Thieme 2005, illustration by Karl Wesker.)

Table 2.2 Summary of somatic and cutaneous innervation

Somatic/Cutaneous Area	Innervation	Spinal Cord Origin
Pubic bone, mons pubis	Iliohyogastric nerve	L1
Mons pubis, anterior labia majora, medial thigh	Ilioinguinal nerve	L1
Lateral thigh from buttocks to anterior thigh	Lateral cutaneous nerve	L2 and L3
Quadriceps femoris, sartorious, and pectineus muscles, medial and anterior thigh	Femoral nerve	L2 to L4
Upper anterior thigh and mons pubis	Genitofemoral nerve	L1 and L2
Adductor muscles and medial aspect of thighs	Obturator nerve	L2 to L4
Levator ani, obturator internus, coccygeous, piriformis, gemelli, and quadratus femoris muscles Buttocks and hip, hamstring and gastrocnemius muscles and lateral lower leg Rectum, levator ani muscles, urogenital triangle, clitoris, vulva	Sacral plexus Sciatic nerve Pudendal nerve	L4 and L5 S1 to S3

Clinical Note

Keep ▶ Fig. 2.35 in mind when reading the concepts of peripheral sensitization.

2.14.1 Pelvic Neuroanatomy[3,4,13,27,28]

The lumbosacral spine receives sensory input from the pelvic, hypogastric, and pudendal nerves. This information is relayed to the dorsal horn and medial/central/lateral gray matter of the lumbosacral spinal cord. Interneurons found within the central gray region of the spinal cord and intermediolateral cell columns of the lumbosacral segments further communicate information. Ascending sensory tracts (spinothalamic dorsal columns and spinoreticular lateral columns) function to relay information to the supraspinal centers of the thalamus and brain stem.

Pelvic efferents and interneurons of the lumbosacral spinal cord reflexes originate in the brain stem and include the nucleus paragigantocellularis, raphe nuclei pallidus, and locus caeruleus. The periaqueductal gray (PAG) matter of the midbrain is heavily interconnected with the brain stem and hypothalamic sites related to sexual behavior, and they have a dual role in both descending modulation of pain, and as a relay station for ascending pain as information travels to the midbrain (mesencephalon).

Clinical Note

Genitalia are innervated by two sets of primary afferent fibers projecting to two distinct regions of neuroaxis:
- Pelvic nerve (S2–4)
  ○ Symptoms from external genitalia
  ○ Lower one-third of vagina and rectum
- Splanchnic nerves (T5 to L2) via hypogastric plexus
  ○ Symptoms from internal genitalia
  ○ Upper two-thirds of vagina and rectum

The visceral nervous system has corresponding efferent branches (ANS) and afferent branches. The efferent system (autonomic) is the motor system of the visceral smooth muscles and glands and consists of sympathetic and parasympathetic fibers supplying the urethra, bladder, ureters, vagina, cervix, uterus, tubes, ovaries, sigmoid colon, rectum, anal canal, visceral peritoneum, and the local vasculature. The afferent system transmits noxious stimuli and other sensations from the abdominal wall, pelvic viscera, and visceral peritoneum to the spinal cord. The viscera and visceral peritoneum initiates painful sensation when stretched, overdistended, or ischemic or when their visceral muscles spasm.

2.15 Pelvic Pain and Nociception

Pain, as defined by the International Association for the Study of Pain, is: "an unpleasant sensory *and* emotional experience that is associated with actual or potential tissue damage or described in such terms." It is instructive to note that pain is always subjective, and that the examiner will find it difficult to interpret whether the patient is experiencing discomfort, pain, or distress. Further complicating this dynamic when discussing the patient's pelvic pain, is that visceral and pelvic pain, unlike somatic pain, does not accurately reflect the degree of tissue damage.

Learning Objectives

- The clinician will describe the differences between central and peripheral sensitization.
- The clinician will discuss the role of cross-system effect as it relates to the patient suffering with a pelvic pain.
- The clinician will identify from which segment of the neuroaxis the patient's pain is originating.

Nociception is defined as the physiological response to tissue damage or a precursor to tissue damage. There are two types of pain receptors that are activated by nociceptive input, low-threshold nociceptors that are typically associated with fast (myelinated) A-delta pain fibers leading to pricking pain, and high-threshold nociceptors that are associated with slow (unmyelinated) C-fibers, resulting in burning or dull pain. The tissue type, when stimulated, will also have an effect on the perceived noxious stimuli. Nerve nociceptors of muscles when stimulated by electrical current will produce an aching pain sensation, whereas those of the viscera will result in vague sensations of "fullness and nausea." It is not until greater intensities of electrical stimulation are applied that the viscera will experience a sensation of pain.[33] Supraspinal regions that include the thalamus, anterior cingulate cortex (ACC), insular cortex (IC), and somatosensory cortex receive visceral nociception via synaptic transmissions from the dorsal horn, and the neurotransmitters, including glutamate, substance P, and N-methyl-D-aspartic acid (NMDA), modulate their postsynaptic responses. Pain can also result from the activation of the central nociceptive pathway in the absence of peripheral nociceptive activation. This is known as central pain. Central pain is commonly associated with motivational-affective pathways that mimic the perception and realization of pain, commonly associated with anxiety, neurosis, depression, and hysteria.[33]

Under normal circumstances nociceptors are inactive and unresponsive and are known as silent nociceptors. Local inflammation will activate these receptors leading to an awakened state causing spontaneous discharges and heightened awareness to peripheral stimulation. These silent nociceptors are found in the nerves of the joints, epithelial cells, and viscera. The degree to which they become responsive to pain is directly proportional to the degree of local inflammation and inflammatory mediator release of bradykinin, prostaglandins, serotonin, and histamine. Tissue injury leads to the activation of these silent nociceptors, receptors that lay dormant in each tissue of one's body; the greater the stimulation, the greater the sensitivity, resulting in hyperalgesia. Hyperalgesia is an elevation of pain to a noxious stimulus after a tissue has been injured, where continued stimulation will lead to a greater amount of pain experienced regardless of whether or not the stimuli is of similar, lesser, or greater magnitude. To this degree, the affected tissue may even be respondent to stimuli that under normal circumstances is nonnoxious. This is known as allodynia.

Allodynia, the experience of intolerable pain from nonnoxious stimuli, is due to the upregulation of neuropeptides, including galanin and vasoactive intestinal polypeptide in the DRG and their central branches, leading to a downregulation of substance P, somatostatin, and calcitonin gene-related peptide. Further damage to Schwann cells will lead to an increased production of messenger ribonucleic acid (RNA) for neurotrophins and their receptors that results in the ingrowth of sympathetic postganglionic axons into the DRG, which leads to an encirclement of their cell bodies. Additionally, peripheral nerve injuries to the large myelinated afferents lead to ingrowth into lamina II. The combination of the two contributes to the formation of allodynia.[33]

Wind-up is the term that defines the temporal summation of repetitive noxious stimulation of the CNS, and it is typically noted as a progressive pain by the suffering patient and is mediated by multiple factors, including: histamine, bradykinin, tumor necrosis factor, prostaglandins, epinephrine, adenosine, nerve growth factor (NGF), and serotonin.[34] Wind-up is thought to be due to peripheral C-fiber nociceptive input, and it is an example of central sensitization occurring at the dorsal horn. Persistent input activates the NMDA and substance-P receptors leading to central hyperalgesia mediated at the spinal cord.[35] Wind-up is best monitored in humans as an increased expression of pain per unit of nociception and when compared with the standard nociceptive reactivity of the uninjured subject.[35,36]

Primary hyperalgesia is the term that is associated with a change in behavior of the nociceptors at the site of injury, and it is experienced at the site of the lesion; whereas secondary hyperalgesia is associated with a change of behavior in the neurons of the central nervous system and is experienced at a location removed from the original injury; nociception can result from mechanical, thermal, or chemical stimulation.[28,33,35] This change in central neurons is directly related to the release of neural mediators, including: prostaglandins, amines, cytokines, kinins, and peptides, which serve to increase the excitability of the CNS, or secondary hyperalgesia.

This "second pain" reflects an increased excitability of spinal cord neurons that is related to central sensitization[37,38,39] and is noted as being duller in nature, often related to the presence of chronic pain. It is believed to be transmitted along the dorsal horn through C-fibers as a result of NMDA activation of second order neurons. The NMDA activation induces calcium entry into the dorsal horn neurons. This activates nitric oxide synthase, which synthesizes nitric oxide, which releases sensory neuropeptides, especially substance-P, resulting in a lower threshold to excitability, and the activation of silent interspinal synapses and the sensitization of second order spinal neurons.[29,30]

Substance-P is known to have long-reaching effects, and it is the likely cause of sensitization of dorsal horns proximally and distally to the initial input locus, resulting in an expansion of receptive fields and the activation of wide dynamic neurons by nonnociceptive afferent impulses. Laboratory experiments have shown that wind-up will occur if a nociceptive stimulus is applied to an affected region more often than once every 3 seconds.[29,30] Neurogenic inflammation, a characteristic of wind-up, is found to occur in both the peripheral nervous system and the CNS. Neurogenic inflammation in the pelvis is primarily mediated through calcitonin gene-related peptide and substance P, and each is highly noted in the afferent neurons of the urinary bladder, distal colon, and reproductive organs.[40] Experimental induction of prostatitis/cystitis demonstrates evidence of progressive mast cell degranulation, and sensory neuropeptide calcitonin gene-related peptides are noted. A resultant product released from these activated mast cells is NGF. NGF is one of the few factors that correlate with pelvic pain.[41,42,43,44] C-fiber sensitization, as a result of neurogenic inflammation, is a product of this NGF being released. NGF is also responsible for the increased production of neuropeptides such as substance P and calcitonin related gene-related peptide when it binds to the receptors on sensory neurons.[41,42,43,44] Persistent activation of silent C-fibers from the viscera of the pelvis results in an increase in noxious input to the dorsal horn. The resulting biochemical changes that result in allodynia and a state of greater neuropathic output. The resulting cascade of events includes neurogenic inflammation, and hypertonicity of the pelvic floor and abdominal musculature.[45,46] A persistence of this noxious stimulation will result in an expansion of the receptor fields, and facilitate pain persistence and sensitization.

Central sensitization is defined as an increased response to stimulation that is mediated by amplification of signaling in the CNS. Although the stimulation does not necessarily need to be of noxious intensity for central sensitization to be present, it should recruit mechanisms that would signal a noxious response. Central sensitization is due to *plastic deformation* of the dorsal horn as a response to the repetitive or sustained noxious stimulus.[34,36,40,42,43,44,47]

Clinical Note

Understanding plastic deformation plays a critical role in the evaluation and treatment of the patient with pelvic pain.

An example of central sensitization is noted with patients suffering from irritable bowel syndrome. They have been found to demonstrate aberrant brain activation patterns during both noxious rectal stimulation and in anticipation of rectal pain.[41,42,43,44] Central sensitization is influenced by forebrain activity as well, where emotions and cognitions can effectively sensitize the spinal cord pain pathway neurons. The end result is a persistent expression of symptoms that become reinforced by chronic activity avoidance, as well as resultant physical deconditioning.[34,48,49]

Further increases of pain are found to occur through the disruption of inhibitory mediators such as the rostroventromedial medulla (RVM) via the PAG, through excessive conscious attention and perseveration; the RVM and PAG are descending, inhibitory tracts that run along the dorsolateral funiculus and are heavily influenced by cognition, emotions, and pain behaviors due to the involvement of the anterior cingulate cortex.[41,42,43,44] This neuroplasticity and resultant CNS hypersensitivity alter the chemical, electrophysiological, and pharmacological systems leading to hyperalgesia and allodynia.+

A unique characteristic of visceral pain is that the severity of injury or insult does not accurately denote the magnitude of the condition, unlike the somatic structures. It is common for visceral pain to be poorly localized, referring to the body wall and accompanied by heightened motor and autonomic reflexes.[29,30] Visceral pain is due to distension, impaction, ischemic, inflammatory, and mesentery traction events, while being insensitive to cutting and burning stimuli.

The viscera, unlike the somatic structures, are innervated by two sets of primary afferent fibers that project to two distinct regions of the neuroaxis. Pelvic nerve afferent fibers originate in the lumbosacral DRG, and project centrally to the sacral spine, whereas the splanchnic nerves project to the T5 to L2 segments of the spinal cord through the hypogastric plexus. Stimulation of the external genitals is carried by the sacral afferent parasympathetic system, whereas the stimulation of the internal genitals is carried by the hypogastric, pelvic, and vagus nerves containing sensory fibers that convey information from the uterus and vagina.[50]

Visceral afferents terminate in lamina I, II, V, and X, and account for 10% of all the afferent inflow. Visceral hyperalgesia is due to inflammation and/or repeated stimulation of a viscous, likely due to the release of NMDA, an amino acid that acts as an agonist, thus mimicking the excitatory action of the neurotransmitter glutamate. Viscera-somatic hyperalgesia is the allogeneic process of a viscous-determining somatic hyperalgesia in an area of referred pain likely due to the convergence of both visceral and somatic afferent fibers on the same neurons of the CNS. The brain will typically refer to the symptoms somatically as there are typically greater experiences of somatic versus visceral pain.[29,30,51,52] Rat studies have demonstrated actual changes in the dorsal horn neurons that have received persistent input from hyperalgesic muscles,[30,51,52] plastic deformation. This can be manifested and inferred in humans as the persistence of symptoms beyond the alleviation of the insulting, painful event.

Clinical Note

There is a mechanical change within the dorsal horn as a result of persistent, noxious stimulation. This leads to the experience of extraordinary symptoms that often do not match the provocative stimulus.

In Chapter 5, strategies are outlined to reverse these plastic changes within the dorsal horn.

Viscera-visceral cross-talk/convergence is an allogeneic condition of a viscous rendering clinical hyperalgesia to another viscous that shares, at least partially, segmental innervation. The convergence of impulses arriving in the spinal cord via visceral afferent fibers in sympathetic nerves creates an unpleasant visceral sensation, initiating a widespread somatic and visceral motor activity, resulting in a sensory experience that is diffuse, poorly localized, and often referred to as a somatic structure. This often results in an increased visceral motility, increased internal secretion, and prolonged muscle spasms. Forty to 60% of all neurons in the lower thoracic segments of the spinal cord receive convergent somatic and visceral input, both of which are typically nociceptive in nature.[53] This phenomenon is noted clinically in the patient suffering from chronic pelvic pain as often having vague, diffuse symptoms that involve structurally unique systems: urogenital, gastrointestinal, and musculoskeletal. This may be explained by the presence of unmyelinated or poorly myelinated nerve fibers from both the viscera and somatic structures, and the spinal cord.[31,53]

Multiple studies have demonstrated female viscera-visceral interactions at T10 to L1 innervations.[29,30,51,52,54,55,56] Examples of cross-system effects would include: bladder inflammation, which reduces the rate of uterine contractions and the effects of drugs on the uterus; and colon inflammation, which produces signs of inflammation in an otherwise healthy bladder and reduces volume voiding thresholds of the bladder.[34,40,57,58,59,60] "The percentage of neurons in the spinal cord which receive convergent input from two or more pelvic organs appears to be higher than the proportion of DRG cells innervating multiple viscera. For example, 26 percent of all recorded neurons in the dorsal horn of lumbo-sacral segments of the spinal cord receive afferent inputs from both the colon and urinary bladder."[40] Intrareferral patterns have been seen between the vestibule, urethra, and bladder of pelvic pain patients as these organs have a common embryological origin.[61,62,63]

Peripheral sensitization, enhancement of the peripheral nervous system, is due to the presence of prolonged, local inflammation or tissue injury, resulting in chronic hyperalgesia of visceral afferents. The sensitized region responds to what had otherwise been innocuous due to the activation of silent receptors. Inflammatory mediators are released and reduce the receptor local firing threshold, thus promoting the transmission of noxious stimuli; peripheral sensitization can persist long after the offending stimulating event. Of clinical importance is that there are more epidermal stem cells in the skin from the scalp, mons

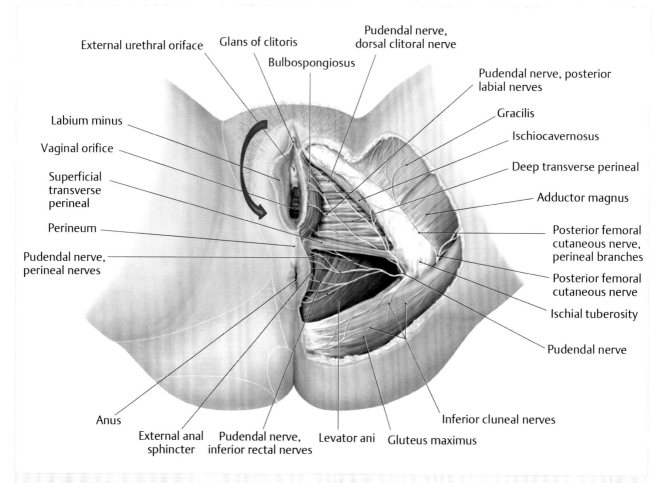

External urethral oriface
Glans of clitoris
Bulbospongiosus
Pudendal nerve, dorsal clitoral nerve
Pudendal nerve, posterior labial nerves
Labium minus
Gracilis
Ischiocavernosus
Vaginal orifice
Superficial transverse perineal
Deep transverse perineal
Adductor magnus
Perineum
Posterior femoral cutaneous nerve, perineal branches
Pudendal nerve, perineal nerves
Posterior femoral cutaneous nerve
Ischial tuberosity
Pudendal nerve
Anus
Inferior cluneal nerves
External anal sphincter
Pudendal nerve, inferior rectal nerves
Levator ani
Gluteus maximus

Fig. 2.36 Example of peripheral sensitization. (From THIEME Atlas of Anatomy, General Anatomy and Musculoskeletal System, © Thieme 2005, illustration by Karl Wesker.)

pubis, and scrotum than other parts of the body,[64,65,66] leading to more pronounced sensation when compared with others that receive exactly the same stimuli, due to this abundance of sensory nerves. This was further confirmed by Tympanidis et al as they found a statistically significant increase in density and number of protein gene product PGP 9.5 immunoreactive cells in the papillary dermis of patients with vulvodynia as compared with a control group.[66]

Clinical Note

Three principal peripheral nociceptors are the:[3,4]
- A-delta mechanical nociceptors, which respond to noxious mechanical stimuli that damage or threaten to damage tissue.
- C-polymodal nociceptors, which respond to noxious mechanical, noxious thermal (> 44°C), and noxious chemical stimuli.
- Silent (or sleeping) nociceptors, which do not respond to acute noxious stimulation of uninjured tissue but become active after tissue is injured.

Information from peripheral nociceptors is conveyed by sensory axons, whose cell bodies are in the DRG, to the spinal cord where they synapse onto second-order spinal cord neurons, which transmit the information to supraspinal sites (▶ Fig. 2.36).

Clinical Note

Recall ▶ Fig. 2.36 and the various peripheral nerves that innervate the pelvic region.

Consider the concept of peripheral sensitization. If the patient experienced persistent irritation to L1, leading to pain along the dermatome outlined by the ilioinguinal nerve, there may be a spill-over effect to the region of dermis typically associated with the pudendal nerve.

Appropriate treatment, in this scenario, would be directed at L1 and not S1–3 as would be the case if the pudendal nerve were to be accountable.

2.15.1 Summary

Pelvic pain, to a great degree, is a result of neurogenic inflammation of the peripheral nervous system and the CNS. This premise is a pivotal concept for the clinician treating the patient with pelvic pain.[36,41,42,43] The consequences of central sensitization, peripheral sensitization, and cross-talk/convergence are necessary for the clinician to understand to provide the best possible treatment approach.

2.16 Functional Integration

The following provides a means in which the clinician will have the opportunity to appreciate the complexity of pelvic neuroanatomy and musculature.

Urine continence is maintained by the elastic fibers of the urethra at the base of the bladder and through the continuous contraction of the sphincter urethrae muscle of the urogenital diaphragm, perineal nerve S2–4. The sensation of "fullness" typically occurs at 250 mL of urine, or 50% of maximal capacity. The full bladder reflex occurs when the receptors sensitive to stretch within the bladder are activated, and afferent fibers of the pelvic splanchnic nerves S2–4 are activated. The result is a stimulation of the smooth musculature of the detrusor muscle, widening and shortening of the urethra at the base of the bladder, and a relaxation of the pubovesicle fibers of the levator ani musculature.[3,4,13]

Conscious control of micturition occurs through branches of the perineal nerve S2–4. With micturition, the sphincter urethra relaxes and the detrusor muscle, abdominal muscles, and respiratory diaphragm increase intraabdominal pressure resulting in the expulsion of urine. In males, the contraction of the bulbospongiosus muscle will assist in the evacuation of remnant urine in the urethra.

Upon completion of urination, sympathetic activity through the hypogastric plexus (T11 to L1) and/or sacral splanchnic nerves (S2–4) relaxes the detrusor muscle, constricting the urethra, and increasing the muscle activity of the pelvic diaphragm and sphincter urethrae to allow refilling of the bladder.

> **Clinical Note**
>
> Peripheral sensitization of the bladder, i.e., interstitial cystitis, is often readily treated at the spinal segments T11, 12 and L1.

There are four components of sexual excitation of the penis or clitoris. These components are sensory, psychological, learned, and environmental. The sensory and psychological aspects will be highlighted to demonstrate the interaction of the peripheral nervous system and the CNS. Sensory components include tactile stimulation of the genital organs resulting in reflexive erection that is inclusive of somatic and parasympathetic systems. The psychological aspect of excitation appears to be more critical in the propagation of sexual excitation. Patients suffering from lower motor neuron injuries are unable to experience sexual excitation with physical stimulation; however, mental imagery will often provide the desired state of arousal, this holds true for those with upper motor neuron lesions as well.[3,4,13]

The pelvic splanchnic nerves (S2–4) are reflexively activated with erotic thoughts or direct stimulation of the genitals resulting in an activation of the parasympathetic nervous system resulting in a relaxation of the smooth muscle fibers within the cavernous erectile tissue of the penis or clitoris with a resultant increase of local acceptance of blood flow to the region.

Concurrently, a contraction of the bulbospongiosus and ischiocavernosus muscles via the perineal nerve (S2–4) limits the outflow from the cavernous spaces resulting in engorgement of these spaces and the presence of an erect penis or clitoris. Resolution, or detumescence, is the return of the penis and clitoris to the flaccid state. This is a result of a contraction of smooth muscles of the spongy tissue restricting the inflow of blood. The contraction of these muscles is stimulated by sympathetic fibers of the cavernous nerves (T10 to L2) and a relaxation of the bulbospongiosus and ischiocavernosus muscles (S2–4).[3,4]

2.17 Anatomy, Lower Urinary Tract

Sensory innervation of the bladder and urethra originates at S2–4, and travels via the parasympathetic pelvic nerve.[3,4] Additional afferents originate in the ganglia of the thoracolumbar levels T11–12 of the sympathetic outflow via the hypogastric nerve. The sensory axons of striated muscle of the external urethral sphincter travel in the somatic pudendal nerve to the sacral region of the spinal cord. Sensory nerves supplying the bladder are either thin myelinated type A-delta or unmyelinated C-fibers. The abdominal viscera is typically insensitive to mechanical pain; however, ischemic events can provoke pain. Referred pain from the bladder is either in the perineal region or suprapubically.

2.18 Biopsychology of Pain

Pain is a complex, highly subjective experience that involves the interaction of three dimensions: sensory-discriminative, affective-motivational, and cognitive-evaluative. Each dimension will influence the other, dynamically interacting with the CNS pain matrix, the neurobiological correlate of the subjective pain experience.[67]

Visceral pain's pain matrix is poorly localized and is often referred to other viscera or somatic regions that share common embryological origin. Visceral stimuli are processed in the S2 (the human secondary somatosensory cortex, a region of cerebral cortex lying mostly on the parietal operculum), IC, medial and orbital subdivisions of the prefrontal cortices (PFC) (MPFC, OPFC, respectively); several subdivisions of the ACC are reported as being critical to CNS processing of visceral stimuli. S2 is important for the primary processing of visceral sensation, whereas higher processing occurs elsewhere.[27,28]

Somatic pain's "pain-matrix" involves the lateral thalamus, primary and secondary somatosensory cortices, and the IC, whereas the activation of the posterior parietal cortex and the PFC account for the cognitive-evaluative processing of painful somatic stimuli.[5,67]

The IC is an important visceral sensorimotor region of the brain that integrates both somatic and visceral input from the sensory thalamus and the NTS, central nucleus of the amygdala, and the rostral-ventral subdivision of the ACC indicating that visceral sensation and emotional information are integrated in the anterior IC. Within the PFC, the OPFC and MPFC, both sensory and motor visceral functions are integrated, as is mood. The PFC has extensive reciprocal connections to the amygdale indicating a significant emotional regulation component, and also many connections to the ACC. The ACC lies at the interface

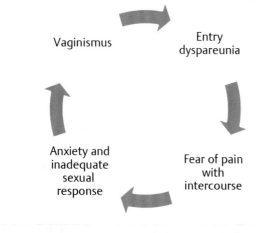

Fig. 2.37 Pain cycle.

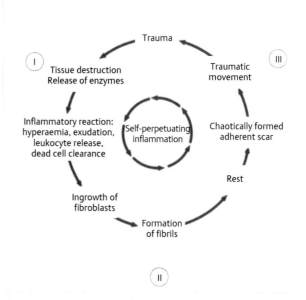

Fig. 2.38 Inflammatory reaction. (From Ombregt L, Bisschop P, ter Veer HJ. A System of Orthopaedic Medicine. 2nd ed. Philadelphia, PA; London: Churchill Livingstone; 2003:1344. Used with permission.)

2.19 Endocrinology, Stress, and Pelvic Pain

Acute and chronic stress has been hypothesized to induce neuroendocrine disturbances and consequent neuroinflammatory stimulus, activating the release of neuropeptides via the hypothalamic-pituitary-adrenal axis, and the ANS. Chronic activation of physiological stress induces putative glucocorticoid resistance and altered immunity, releasing proinflammatory cytokines and prostaglandins that may contribute to pelvic tension myalgia, and cycling/repeating psychological distress.[68]

As noted in ▶ Fig. 2.39, a trauma leads to the inflammatory reaction, which as previously discussed, initiates the myofibril activity that shortens and tightens the fascia of the local region. This tension of the fascia is often experienced as a pressure-pain, which will further limit activity and causes greater fibroblast proliferation, further restricting movement, which then deconditions the body leading to less likelihood of activity thereby cementing the dysfunctional status. The increased pressure-pain experience provides an additional point of painful reference for the patient to focus on selective exaggeration of pain through the PAG.

Patients with chronic conditions including pelvic pain, irritable bowel disease (IBS), and other conditions have a twofold increase in somatic comorbidities when compared with the unaffected population, and a positive correlation between IBS and mood disorder, health anxiety, neuroticism, adverse life events, reduced quality of life, and increased health care seeking behaviors.

Increased sympathetic activity and a decrease in parasympathetic activity have been found in those patients suffering from chronic pain conditions including fibromyalgia, IBS, migraines, and pelvic pain. Of those suffering from chronic

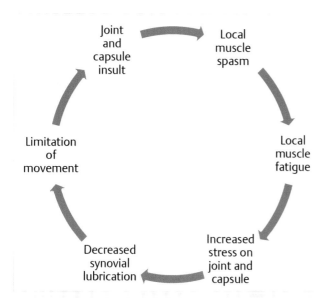

Fig. 2.39 Muscle spasm and pain cycle. (From Howard FM, ed. Pelvic Pain; Diagnosis & Management. Philadelphia, Baltimore, New York, London, Buenos Aires, Hong Kong, Sydney & Tokyo: Lippincott Williams & Wilkins; 2000. Used with permission.)

of sensory and emotional processing, and it may be the most important structure involved in emotional state on perception of visceral sensation and/or pain, and vice versa. The ACC provides output to the autonomic structures involved in the regulation of arousal (LC) and to the amygdala. Visceral hypersensitivity, visceral responses, can be conditioned in a classic Pavlovian fashion. Distinct neural circuits generate emotion-specific patterns of autonomic and endocrine output to the body in general, and the viscera specifically.[5]

A common pain cycle is noted in ▶ Fig. 2.37.[68]

pelvic pain, 49.9% also suffer from IBS. Similarities of IBS and fibromyalgia and visceral hypersensitivity and chronic pelvic pain with associated changes in the ANS are noted to share the same splanchnic afferent innervation as the colon and rectum.[69]

It must also be taken into consideration that a woman's tolerance to pain will fluctuate throughout the menstrual cycle. The threshold to pain is less during the perimenstrual phase, and highest during the luteal phase. This is especially noted along the abdomen of those suffering from dysmenorrhea. The symptoms may last beyond the cessation of menses.

2.20 Pathology

2.20.1 Musculotendinous Pathoanatomy

Injuries to the hip and pelvis are characterized as either macrotraumatic or microtraumatic. Acute macrotrauma to the pelvis commonly involves the overlying soft tissue and musculotendinous attachments of the pelvis.[9,10] Overuse and/or excessive stresses applied to a musculotendinous structure can induce micro- and macrotrauma. The result is the formation of a scar within the affected muscle belly, at the musculotendinous and/or tenoperiosteal junctions. When evaluating the young athlete, a frank apophyseal avulsion must be considered. Athletic, macrotraumatic fractures or fracture dislocations of the pelvic ring are rare except in equestrian events.[9,10]

Learning Objectives

- The clinician will describe the biomechanical mechanisms to which the pelvic ring and pelvis can be afflicted.
- The clinician will discriminate between the various pathologies of the pelvic ring and pelvis that may give rise to similar symptoms.
- The clinician will employ unique evaluation strategies to rule in or out various pathologies.

Overuse injuries from repetitive microtraumas of the pelvis are on the increase and can be found along the insertion points along the pelvis.[9,10] Osteitis pubis may present as an adductor strain in those athletes who run on, or participate in sports on hard surfaces including indoor soccer, hockey, tennis, and track and field. Dancers and other athletes who participate in endurance activities are prone to develop a "snapping hip" that is typically either an iliotibial band syndrome or the tendinous glide of the iliopsoas over the neck of the femur[9,10] as a result of a sustained tension through the muscle-tendon unit passing over a bony prominence.

Repetitive stress injuries can be voluntary or involuntary alike. Voluntary repetitive maneuvers such as those seen in sporting or vocational activities that require sustained or repeated movements account for a multitude of injuries that adversely affect the musculotendinous units as a result of the persistent, repetitive load to which the musculotendinous structures undergo. This is a common finding in the musculotendinous structures of the pelvis, and one that is on the increase among the adolescent population.[9,10] The patient suffering from pelvic pain, however, may undergo an involuntary repetitive musculotendinous loading. In a fashion that is similar

to bruxing in the dental field (clinching the muscles of mastication), the patient suffering from pelvic pain will often demonstrate greater resting tone of the pelvic floor musculature during common activities of daily living. With this concept in mind, it is important to consider when evaluating the patient with pelvic pain that with a constant load and repeated stress, the formation of a tendinopathy is conceivable.

Pelvic Bruxing?

Pelvic bruxing is analogous to temporomandibular joint (TMJ) bruxing. Commonalities between the patient suffering with pelvic pain, and TMJ pain are: increased anxiety, stress sensitive, and depression. As the muscles of mastication are adversely impacted as a result of constant grinding of the teeth, so too are the pelvic muscles negatively impacted by a persistent state of contraction and hypertonicity.

Healthy tendons consist of dense, clearly defined, parallel collagen bundles with a supply of arteries that are oriented parallel to the collagen fibers in the endotenon. Tendinopathy is used as a generic descriptor to include all pathologies that arise from and around tendons including tendinitis, tendinosis, and paratendinitis. These conditions are characterized by pain and soreness along the tendon, increased proteoglycan content, collagen disorganization, cellular changes, and neurovascular ingrowths.[70,71] A tendinopathy will demonstrate degeneration and a disordered arrangement of collagen fibers, an increased vascularity that is found at right angles to the collagen fibers, and collagen degeneration and loss of parallel orientation. A tendinosis is tendon degeneration without clinical or histological signs of an inflammatory response.[72,73,74,75] Collagen degeneration, fiber disorientation, and an increased mucoid extracellular matrix in the absence of inflammatory cells are the primary histopathological characteristics of tendinopathies. The degree to which a lesion presents itself will vary depending on the specific locality of the lesion, and the causative insult.

The tendinopathy cycle begins when the breakdown process exceeds the reparative process due to prolonged stresses and demands being placed upon the tissue, although it is not uncommon for patients to have a clear recollection of a specific mechanism or moment of onset.[70,73,74] After tissue damage, the reparation process begins, and as noted above results in tissue of lesser quality. The excessive Type III collagen formation when compared with Type I collagen results in tissue that is less organized with regards to the appropriate parallel structure, decreasing the tensile strength to linear loads, and making it more susceptible to re-injury. Repeated stresses further the accumulation of inferior collagen deposits, resulting in a more globally weakened tissue that is more vulnerable to injury. Both conscious and unconscious restriction of activities will further decondition the affected muscle. This increases the likelihood of re-injury and chronic tendinopathies.

Clinical Note

The resultant disorganization of collagen fibers after an injury is the theoretical foundation for transverse friction massage as a treatment.

Clinical Note

A tendinosis suggests the presence of degenerative pathology in the absence of an active inflammation, resulting in chronic tendon injuries. The pain associated with a tendinosis is due to the accumulation of microtraumas and a failure to completely heal, and not to inflammation.

The pain from tendinopathy is due to the mechanical separation of collagen fibers and disruption of tissue integrity, in addition to the release of noninflammatory biochemical substances such as glycosamines, especially chondroitin sulphate.[70,73]

Patients with chronic tendinopathies may have complaints of tingling or numbness distal to the lesion due to the thickening of the muscle tendon unit leading to a compromise of neural mobility. The local inflammation of the musculoskeletal unit will further compromise the local nerve mobility resulting in a local neuritis.[70,73]

The degree to which the tendinopathy affects the patient is largely dependent upon multiple factors including:
• The degree of overuse and lack of recovery time
• The individual's genetics
• Ergonomics associated with common activities of daily living
• The individual's age, fitness level, and general health
• The duration of injury prior to treatment initiation
• The quality of medical care/advice received[70,75]

The healing tendon tissue is often deficient in tensile strength frequently being 30% lower than the unaffected side. This deficit can last for months to years following an injury. Normal healing begins with the deposition of a greater concentration of Type III collagen, rather than Type I, with appropriate composition returning over time in the absence of trauma. When considering the patient with pelvic pain, and the common splinting/bracing proclivities of the hip and pelvic floor musculature, it is probable that full healing will never be attained and the patient will not get past the initial phase of healing, resulting in a tissue that is more fragile and susceptible to irritation. Poor healing may also be attributable to the persistent exposure to NGF, which promotes the formation of abnormal collagen which, given chronic repetitive irritation, may become permanent even after the exposure to NGF ceases.[41,42,44,47] Gender also plays a role in the formation of a tendinopathy; women are more susceptible to chronic overuse injuries and studies have found a lesser quantity of collagen in the female tendons and a greater Type III to Type I ratio.[45,46]

As previously mentioned, pelvic avulsion injuries occur in both the young and the active mature person; however, they are more common in the skeletally immature population. Typically, avulsion injuries occur as a result of a single violent movement or a combination of lower-load microtraumas at the unfused apophysis at the level of the tendinous insertion; analogous to a common musculotendinous injury in the skeletally mature. Avulsion injuries to the pelvis are common in the skeletally immature due to the inherent weakness along the unfused apophysis, and result in a separation and retraction of the partially ossified apophysis.[17,18] Apophyseal injures typically result from a violent forceful contraction of the respective muscle, and are commonly associated with jumping, sprinting, or running.

The ischial tuberosity is the most common location for apophyseal avulsion injury in the pelvis and is typically due to a forceful contraction of the hamstring musculature, often associated with sprinting or excessive lengthening, as commonly occurs during cheerleading or gymnastics. There may be a sensation of popping at the time of the injury, which often presents itself as severe pain along the posterior thigh and gluteal region. Often there is a compromised gait that accompanies the injury. The ischial tuberosity is the site of origin of the semimembranosus, semitendinosus, adductor magnus, and the long head of the biceps femoris tendon apophysis.[17,18] Radiographic imaging may demonstrate a fracture fragment > 2 cm, which may lead to a fibrous union. Chronic avulsion injuries often lead to extensive callus formation and the resultant heterotopic bone formation may be noted on radiographic assessment.[18] The sciatic nerve runs in close proximity, and its mobility may be compromised in association with hamstring avulsion injuries, and this is to be considered in the young athlete who is unable to touch her toes during forward flexion.[18]

The ASIS is the site of origin of the sartorius tendon and the tensor muscle of the fascia latae. Avulsion injuries often occur here in sprinters during forceful extension of the hip with concurrent knee flexion. Local avulsions at the ASIS are typically less debilitating than those of the ischial tuberosity.[18]

The anterior inferior iliac spine (AIIS) is the site of origin of the rectus femoris tendon, and injuries to it often occur as a result of forceful eccentric hip extension. The most common region of avulsion is noted to be proximal and lateral to the acetabular rim, measuring < 2 cm in size, making it difficult to detect with standard anteroposterior radiographic imaging. Oblique views may more appropriately demonstrate local injuries of this nature. Chronic injuries may lead to heterotopic bone formation.[18]

The anterior iliac crest is the site of the attachment of the abdominal musculature, and avulsion injuries occurring along this region in the adolescent population have been noted in those 18 years of age and younger. The typical mechanism of injury is associated with running or jumping, but it may also occur as a result of direct trauma.[18] Bilateral symptomatic iliac crest apophyseal avulsions are not uncommon in the young athletic population and may create confusion when bilateral radiographic comparisons are made.[18]

The pubic symphysis and inferior pubic ramus are the insertion points of the distal attachment of the levator ani and rectus abdominis muscles and are the sites of origin of the adductors of the hip: the adductors longus, brevis, and gracilis. Avulsion injuries are associated with repetitive stress as a result of excessive twisting and turning movements of the abdomen and pelvis, as seen in soccer, ice hockey, and tennis athletes. Often referred to as "athletica pubalgia," there are other pathologies that must be ruled out by the clinician including: osteitis pubis, sportsman's hernia, acetabular labral tears of the hip, sacroiliitis, and lumbar diskogenic disease.[18] Avulsion injuries of the pubic symphysis rarely result in bony displacement and are typically noted as an isolated soft-tissue injury.[18] Radiographic examination may demonstrate sclerosis of the pubic symphysis in the chronically injured. MRI typically demonstrates bone marrow edema at the site of the adductor attachment.[18]

Clinical Note

Considering that the pubic symphysis matures at approximately 18 years of age in the female population, and the heightened physical activity level for youth, it is becoming more common to find remnants of avulsion injuries in the adult population suffering with pelvic pain; bony irregularities along the posterior aspect of the pubic bone are very common.

The lesser trochanter is the insertion of the iliopsoas tendon. Avulsions here are rare, but are sometimes seen in soccer as a result of a forceful contraction of the iliopsoas while the thigh is fixed in an extended position when a player is hit by another while kicking the ball.[18] MRI may demonstrate edema within the growth plate and bone marrow within the apophysis. Older injuries may demonstrate heterotopic bone formation, which may be viewed on X-ray and can often be palpated.

Avulsion injuries can also be present in the adult athlete, and are typically associated with an increased activity level that can be relieved with rest. This patient will present with groin or medial thigh pain as a result of repetitive avulsive or traction forces along the medial aspect of the femur at the level of the insertion of the adductor longus and brevis tendons. The pain will often be diffuse and vague, and confirmation with clinical testing may be difficult to illicit in the patient. The injury is typically associated with long-distance runners and female military recruits.[18] Adductor avulsion syndrome is noted in the literature as "thigh splints." Lesser trochanteric avulsions and avulsions of the pubic symphysis in the adult are to be considered red flags for serious pathology. Nontraumatic avulsions in the adult pelvis should raise concern for a pathological fracture and are often a result of metastatic disease.[18]

2.20.2 Atrophy

Muscle unloading results in a loss of muscle mass and occurs when the supportive, or locomotive functions are not maintained. The extent to which muscle loss occurs is dependent on the degree to which the muscle itself is unloaded. Atrophy, unloading induced atrophy, is considered to be an uncomplicated form of muscle loss due to the loss of mechanical input.[76] In vivo measurements of human muscle protein turnover in disuse indicate that the primary variable of change is a loss of protein synthesis, which is reduced in both the postabsorptive and postprandial states; excessive proteolysis is not evident. The proteolysis becomes dominant by default, but not enhanced. Both Type I and Type II collagen fibers demonstrate equal rate of loss.[76]

This becomes an important concept as it relates to the patient suffering with pelvic pain. All too often this population significantly limits their activity of daily living in an attempt to minimize their pain. The resultant functional weakness further predisposes the patient to greater joint loading and compressive injuries to the chondral structures of the joints of the spine and coxofemoral joint with resultant inflammatory response and symptom aggravation.

2.20.3 Muscle Tenderness and Trigger Points

The clinician must differentiate between muscle tenderness and trigger points.[77] Distinguishing between trigger points and myalgic tender points is necessary when diagnosing a patient. It has been found that one must assess, and when appropriate, provide a mobilization/manipulation examination to not only the immediate joint, but also to those above the affected muscle. After assuring appropriate joint movement, osteokinematically and arthrokinematically, if a taut band persists and it demonstrates the characteristic "twitch" and it demonstrates a predictable referral pattern of pain, only then may it accurately be labeled a trigger point.[1,78]

The motor end plate has been implicated as a central etiological factor with myofascial trigger points, whereas fibromyalgia tender points do not have a motor component. This is confirmed by biopsy where trigger points were found to stain darkly and to demonstrate significantly larger diameter of muscle fibers when compared with normal.[77,78]

2.20.4 Formation of Muscle Spasms Due to Joint Trauma

Both the capsule and ligaments of a joint are pain sensitive structures. Even minor insults can produce pain. Reflexive action to capsular pain is muscle spasm. Spasms, in return, initiate fatigue, which increases joint stress, which can increase capsular and ligamentous stress that will further produce muscular spasms (► Fig. 2.39). Fatigue, pain, and spasms may initiate conscious or subconscious immobilization, which will result in the loss of normal synovial lubrication yielding limited movement, which too can produce spasms. During the early stages of injury, resistance to movement is likely due to spasms set up by nociceptive afferents from Type IV receptors found within the joint tissues. Type IV receptors project polysynaptically to alpha motor neurons and the excitation of the Type IV nociceptive system and pain is perceived as muscle spasm.[79] Persistent muscle activation due to the adaption of stress-related postures may lead to the initiation of tenoperiosteal tendonopathy, which then leads to increased local inflammation and subsequent fascial restrictions. The fascial restrictions, in turn, provoke pain, causing the patient to assume a protective posture (splinting), which minimizes a patient's desire/ability to move, further reducing the local nourishment of the osseous and muscular systems and retarding the healing process, causing greater tissue breakdown resulting in a continuation of the cycle.

2.20.5 Scars

Scars are the normal formation of fibrous tissue formed as a result of tissue damage both internally and externally, traumatic and surgical alike. The resultant tissue is of inferior quality, and demonstrates less tensile strength, 30% less loading capacity in all directions, and less resistance to ultraviolet radiation. Scars, often a result of perpendicular tension being placed along the wound, lead to the excessive proliferation of dermal tissue, with an excessive deposition of fibroblasts from the ECM, especially collagen. Persistent irritation and inflammation will lead to fibrosis, which results in plaque of scar tissue that is raised, rigid, and often red. Often the musculature immediately surrounding a scar is reflexively inhibited, allowing for a local atrophy of the musculature, rendering it more likely to be injured. The subsequent secondary injuries account for the progressive accumulation of inelastic scar tissue, and account for the greater incident rate of complete musculotendinous rupture.[74,80,81,82,83]

Scar maturation begins at week 6 to 8 after epithialization has occurred and continues for 6 to 24 months.[84] Prophylactic treatments are employed to downregulate the persistent synthesis of proinflammatory/fibrogenic cytokines, interluekin-1-beta, tumor necrosis factor-alpha, platelet-derived growth factor, and transforming growth factor-beta.[84]

Symptoms associated with scars are:
- Disfigurement
- Tenderness/pain
- Muscle weakness and inactivation
- Pruritus
- Contractures (loss of motion)
- Sleep disturbances
- Anxiety
- Disruption of daily activities

In both keloid and hypertrophic scar formation there is an excessive accumulation of collagen that may be the result of bacterial infection, skin tension during the healing phase, anoxia, or prolonged inflammatory response. Keloid and hypertrophic scars are noted as an overzealous healing response above the skin where the most significant point of differentiation is that the keloid scar will continue to enlarge beyond the original scope of injury, whereas the hypertrophic scar will typically be limited to the confines of the original injury and may regress spontaneously over time.

As a complex organ derived from two germ layers, the healing of skin is accomplished from the formation of a fibrous tissue plaque.[80] During the normal healing process there is a decrease in cellularity during the transition from granulation tissue to scarring, mediated by apoptosis and the remodeling of the ECM. Widening scars are those that separate during the healing process, often as a result of a perpendicular tension placed along the wound and resulting in hypertrophic scarring. Hypertrophic scars present as a result of persistent irritation and inflammation and lead to fibrotic alterations of cutaneous wound healing and are noted as a proliferation of dermal tissue and an excessive deposition of fibroblasts from the ECM proteins, especially collagen. The result is a plaque of scar tissue that is raised, rigid, and often red.

Studies have shown that hypertrophic scarring is preventable with management of the scar after the wound has healed and full epithelialization has occurred.[84,85] Prophylactic treatment aims at accelerating wound healing by downregulating the persistent synthesis of proinflammatory/fibrogenic cytokines such as interleukin-1-beta, tumor necrosis factor-alpha, platelet-derived growth factor, and transforming growth factor-beta from inflammatory cells. Pressure garments may offer some assistance in scar maintenance; however, the evidence is controversial.[85] Symptoms associated with scarring include disfigurement, tenderness/pain, pruritus, contractures (loss of motion), sleep disturbances, anxiety, depression, and disruption of daily activity.[86]

Perineal trauma is common with spontaneous vaginal deliveries (▶ Fig. 2.40). Perineal trauma during vaginal delivery of primaparas as compared with multiparas is 31 versus 6%.[84]

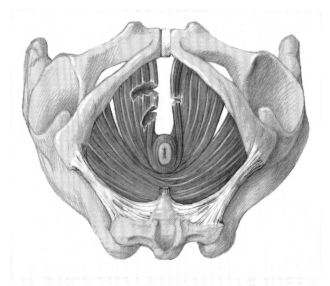

Fig. 2.40 Tearing of puborectalis during spontaneous vaginal delivery. (Adapted from THIEME Atlas of Anatomy, General Anatomy and Musculoskeletal System, © Thieme 2005, illustration by Karl Wesker.)

Those who undergo assisted delivery with the use of forceps, vacuum, and/or episiotomy have an increased likelihood of scar formation and report greater sexual problems, perineal pain, and bowel disturbances than those who had unassisted vaginal deliveries.[84] Adhesions that may cause pelvic pain may be due to endometriosis, pelvic inflammatory disease, trauma, surgery (assisted delivery), and neoplasms. Scars have been implicated as a cause of infertility due to restrictions of tubal mobility or access of ova to tubal fimbriae.[87]

Postoperative scarring is well documented and may be a cause of small bowel obstruction, infertility, and pain, potentially accounting for > 40% of all intestinal obstructions and 60 to 70% involving the small bowel. Adhesions are found in 46% of all cesarean sections, increasing with repeated cesarean sections.[88] A unique characteristic of cesarean sections is the predominance of scar occurring between the uterus, bladder, and omentum due to the presence of amniotic fluid spilling into the upper abdomen, preventing intraabdominal and surgical site adhesions.[88] This compares to surgical procedures directed at the gallbladder, gastric operations, and colectomies that cause abdominal pain, constipation, gastroenterological symptoms, and ileus.[89] Persistent lower back pain and pelvic pain have been associated with elective cesarean sections: the greater the number of cesarean sections the greater the likelihood of developing a pain phenomenon.[90,91] This behavior conflicts with the research conducted by Drew et al, who found no correlation of cesarean section and lower back pain/pelvic pain.[92]

There are four stages of adbominopelvic adhesions that the clinician is to take into consideration[13]
- Stage I: filmy adhesions; nonvascular, easy to release
- Stage II: extensive, nonvascularized, filmy adhesions involving one or more intraabdominal organs
- Stage III: numerous, partially vascularized adhesions involving one or more intraperitoneal organs; may impair function
- Stage IV: as stage III, with dense vascularized adhesions involving the serosa of small bowel or colon, fixed to outer peritoneum

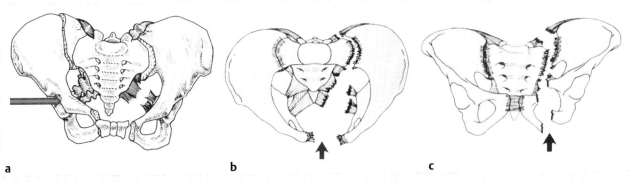

Fig. 2.41 a–c Pelvic trauma classification.

2.20.6 Disk-related Pathoanatomy

Injuries to the disk are characterized as being either primary or secondary in nature. A primary disk lesion is considered when there is typically a single event, or moment that is more rapid in nature that causes the nuclear pulposis to bulge or herniate through the annular shell, more typically noted in the younger population. A secondary disk lesion is that which is associated with repeated stresses, and is considered to be more degenerative in nature; symptoms typically present themselves as a result of aging and/or pathological changes. Structurally, the annulus has sensory nerves along its surface, without penetration to the nucleus. Therefore, it is the disruption of the integrity of the annulus' external surface that provokes pain.[1,2,3,4]

2.20.7 Chondropathy

The ZAJs of the spine are prone to developing degenerative pathology most often in the adult population older than 45 years of age as a result of the degradation of the intervertebral disks. The resultant pain presentation and experience by the patient may be quite similar to that of an intervertebral disk lesion, where active motions of the spine provoke pain that is local or referred. A distinguishing component of an injury to a ZAJ is that motions that induce maximal compression to the ZAJ are most likely to be provocative: extension, side-flexion, and ipsilateral rotation.

2.20.8 SIJ Pathoanatomy

The most common cause for acute sacroiliitis, other than ankylosing spondylitis, is infection. The patient's symptoms will often be unilateral with radiation to the ipsilateral glutei and posterior thigh. All motions that involve the SIJ will be avoided, and feared by the patient, due to the severity of symptoms inclusive of coughing and sneezing. Provocation tests of the SIJ are positive, as are ipsilateral hip motions at end range. Local warmth and edema may be noted, and during a rectal examination the patient will have severe tenderness to palpation of the sacrotuberous, sacrospinous, and anterior SIJ ligaments. Infectious sacroiliitis will demonstrate as above; however, the patient will have a fever and overall general malaise. Blood work will demonstrate high erythrocyte sedimentation rate and leukocytosis. An acute, noninfectious, sacroiliitis is due to local trauma, gout, pyrophosphate, arthropathy, rheumatoid arthritis, osteomyelitis of the ilium, and gluteal abscess. Chronic sacroiliitis is noted when the patient has pain lasting for 3 or more months, and is typically less severe than the acute condition; intermittent exacerbations are noted and it can be quite severe.

Whereas physical therapists often treat the nonsurgical micortrauma of the skeleton and its related structures, medical doctors more often treat the macrotraumatic events. Their research, however, can be utilized as a means of deducting the trauma that a common patient will be seen for at a physical therapist's office. As per the findings of Young-Burgess' 1986 report,[93] pelvic fractures and injuries to the SIJ can occur as a result of lateral compression forces, anterior to posterior compression forces, vertical shear forces, or a combination of forces. The purpose of their research was to determine the effects of macrotrauma to the pelvic ring as related to trauma. In physical therapy, clinicians work with microtrauma to the ligamentous structures. Information, however, can be gleaned from the work of Young-Burgess as it applies to the patient commonly seen in the physical therapy setting suffering from pelvic ring injuries. Subfracture lateral compressive forces occur commonly in athletics where one athlete is tackling another such as in American football and hockey, or during Greco-Roman wrestling. Subfracture anterior-posterior pelvic ring trauma occurs commonly in the patient involved in a sport where there is often a moving body over a fixed leg such as in a kicking motion, or more violently, in skiing injuries (▶ Fig. 2.41).[18]

The most common pelvic fracture occurs as a result of a lateral compression force through the posterior half of the ilium where the force is directed over the anterior half of the iliac wing. This leads to a rotation of the hemipelvis inward with a posterior disruption of the SIJ ligament complex.

Anterior to posterior forces often introduce an external rotation of the hemipelvis, where the pelvis springs open over the intact posterior ligaments as a result of forces being applied to the ASIS; the result is an external rotation of the hemipelvis. Injuries to the bladder, urethra, rectum, and vagina are possible as a result of blunt trauma.

A vertical shear force can lead to a tearing away of the hemipelvis from the sacrum and is typically found as a result of a fall with unilateral landing through the leg or pelvis. This injury typically involves the disruption of the sacrospinous and sacrotuberous ligaments: avulsions in the young and bone fractures in the elderly. Combination injuries are those that involve a combination of vector forces applied to the pelvis; often these are seen in an ejection/landing injury.

2.20.9 Pathology of the Pubic Symphysis

Injuries to the pubic symphysis can be due to the aforementioned mechanisms and should be considered during the course of the evaluation. In addition to the traumatic mechanisms mentioned, complications as a result of pregnancy, as it relates to the pubic symphysis, are estimated be in the range of 1:300. The patient will present with pain and tenderness with radiations to the posterior thigh and demonstrate difficulty in ambulation, and the potential for bladder dysfunction is possible.

References

[1] Cyriax J, Ed. (1982). Textbook of orthopaedic medicine. London, Philadelphia, Toronto, Sydney & Tokyo: WB Saunders & Bailliere Tinda

[2] Ombregt L, Ed. (2003). A system of orthopaedic medicine (2nd ed.). Philadelphia, London: Churchill Livingstone

[3] Larson W, Ed. (2002). Anatomy: Development, function, clinical correlations. Philadelphia, London, New York, St. Louis, Sydney & Toronto: Saunders

[4] Moore KL, Dalley AF, Eds. (2006). Clinically orientated anatomy (5th ed.). Baltimore, Philadelphia: Lippincott Williams & Wilkins

[5] Van Oudenhove L, Demyttenaere K, Tack J, Aziz Q. Central nervous system involvement in functional gastrointestinal disorders. Best Pract Res Clin Gastroenterol 2004; 18: 663–680

[6] Maitland G, Ed. (2005). Maitland's vertebral manipulation. Edinburgh, London, New York, Oxford, Philadelphia, St. Louis, Sydney, Toronto: Elisevier

[7] Jenkins DB, Ed. (2009). Hollinshead's functional anatomy of the limbs and back. Canada: Saunders

[8] Fredberg U, Stengaard-Pedersen K. Chronic tendinopathy tissue pathology, pain mechanisms, and etiology with a special focus on inflammation. Scand J Med Sci Sports 2008; 18: 3–15

[9] Micheli LJ, Smith AD. Sports injuries in children. Curr Probl Pediatr 1982; 12: 1–54

[10] Micheli LJ. Overuse injuries in children's sports: the growth factor. Orthop Clin North Am 1983; 14: 337–360

[11] Schleip R, Klingler W, Lehmann-Horn F. Active fascial contractility: fascia may be able to contract in a smooth muscle-like manner and thereby influence musculoskeletal dynamics. Med Hypotheses 2005; 65: 273–277

[12] Schleip R, Naylor IL, Ursu D et al. Passive muscle stiffness may be influenced by active contractility of intramuscular connective tissue. Med Hypotheses 2006; 66: 66–71

[13] Howard FM, Ed. (2000). Pelvic pain: Diagnosis & management. Philadelphia, Baltimore, New York, London, Buenos Aires, Hong Kong, Sydney & Tokyo: Lippincott Williams & Wilkins

[14] Raoul S, Faure A, Robert R et al. Role of the sinu-vertebral nerve in low back pain and anatomical basis of therapeutic implications. Surg Radiol Anat 2003; 24: 366–371

[15] Maynard LM, Guo SS, Chumlea WC et al. Total-body and regional bone mineral content and areal bone mineral density in children aged 8–18 y: the Fels Longitudinal Study. Am J Clin Nutr 1998; 68: 1111–1117

[16] Nguyen TV, Maynard LM, Towne B et al. Sex differences in bone mass acquisition during growth: the Fels Longitudinal Study. J Clin Densitom 2001; 4: 147–157

[17] Bui-Mansfield LT, Chew FS, Lenchik L, Kline MJ, Boles CA. Nontraumatic avulsions of the pelvis. AJR Am J Roentgenol 2002; 178: 423–427

[18] Sanders TG, Zlatkin MB. Avulsion injuries of the pelvis. Semin Musculoskelet Radiol 2008; 12: 42–53

[19] Burnett RS, Della Rocca GJ, Prather H, Curry M, Maloney WJ, Clohisy JC. Clinical presentation of patients with tears of the acetabular labrum. J Bone Joint Surg Am 2006; 88: 1448–1457

[20] Prather H, Hunt D, Fournie A, Clohisy JC. Early intra-articular hip disease presenting with posterior pelvic and groin pain. PM R 2009; 1: 809–815

[21] Gray H, Bannister LH, Berry MM, Williams PL, Eds. Gray's anatomy: The anatomical basis of medicine & surgery. New York: Churchill Livingston; 1995

[22] Torres M, Gómez-Pardo E, Dressler GR, Gruss P. Pax-2 controls multiple steps of urogenital development. Development 1995; 121: 4057–4065

[23] Mercer S. Anatomy in practice: The ischiorectal fossae. NZ J of Physiotherapy, 2005, 2: 61-64

[24] Levi AC, Borghi F, Garavoglia M. Development of the anal canal muscles. Dis Colon Rectum 1991; 34: 262–266

[25] Barber MD, Bremer RE, Thor KB, Dolber PC, Kuehl TJ, Coates KW. Innervation of the female levator ani muscles. Am J Obstet Gynecol 2002; 187: 64–71

[26] Vleeming A, de Vries HJ, Mens JM, van Wingerden JP. Possible role of the long dorsal sacroiliac ligament in women with peripartum pelvic pain. Acta Obstet Gynecol Scand 2002; 81: 430–436

[27] Haines DE, Ed. Fundamental neuroscience for basic and clinical applications. Philadelphia, New York, London, Buenos Aires, Hong Kong, Sydney, Tokyo: Churchill Livingstone; Elsevier; 2006

[28] Haines DE, Ed. Neuroanatomy: An atlas of structures, sections and systems (7th ed.). Philadelphia, Baltimore, New York, London, Buenos Aires, Hong Kong, Sydney, Tokyo: Wolters Kluwer and Lippincott Williams & Wilkins; 2008

[29] Al-Chaer ED, Lawand NB, Westlund KN, Willis WD. Pelvic visceral input into the nucleus gracilis is largely mediated by the postsynaptic dorsal column pathway. J Neurophysiol 1996; 76: 2675–2690

[30] Al-Chaer ED, Traub RJ. Biological basis of visceral pain: recent developments. Pain 2002; 96: 221–225

[31] Lamvu G, Steege JF. The anatomy and neurophysiology of pelvic pain. J Minim Invasive Gynecol 2006; 13: 516–522

[32] Rogers RM, Jr. Basic neuroanatomy for understanding pelvic pain. J Am Assoc Gynecol Laparosc 1999; 6: 15–29

[33] Willis WD, Westlund KN. Neuroanatomy of the pain system and of the pathways that modulate pain. J Clin Neurophysiol 1997; 14: 2–31

[34] Klumpp DJ, Rudick CN. Summation model of pelvic pain in interstitial cystitis. Nat Clin Pract Urol 2008; 5: 494–500

[35] Price DD, Hayes RL, Ruda M, Dubner R. Spatial and temporal transformations of input to spinothalamic tract neurons and their relation to somatic sensations. J Neurophysiol 1978; 41: 933–947

[36] George SZ, Bishop MD, Bialosky JE, Zeppieri G, Jr, Robinson ME. Immediate effects of spinal manipulation on thermal pain sensitivity: an experimental study. BMC Musculoskelet Disord 2006; 7: 68

[37] Staud R. Evidence of involvement of central neural mechanisms in generating fibromyalgia pain. Curr Rheumatol Rep 2002; 4: 299–305

[38] Staud R, Robinson ME, Vierck CJ, Jr, Cannon RC, Mauderli AP, Price DD. Ratings of experimental pain and pain-related negative affect predict clinical pain in patients with fibromyalgia syndrome. Pain 2003; 105: 215–222

[39] Staud R, Price DD, Robinson ME, Mauderli AP, Vierck CJ. Maintenance of windup of second pain requires less frequent stimulation in fibromyalgia patients compared to normal controls. Pain 2004; 110: 689–696

[40] Malykhina AP. Neural mechanisms of pelvic organ cross-sensitization. Neuroscience 2007; 149: 660–672

[41] Pontari MA, Ruggieri MR. Mechanisms in prostatitis/chronic pelvic pain syndrome. J Urol 2004; 172: 839–845

[42] Pontari MA. Etiologic theories of chronic prostatitis/chronic pelvic pain syndrome. Curr Urol Rep 2007; 8: 307–312

[43] Pontari MA, Ruggieri MR. Mechanisms in prostatitis/chronic pelvic pain syndrome. J Urol 2008; 179 Suppl: S61–S67

[44] Pontari MA. Chronic prostatitis/chronic pelvic pain syndrome. Urol Clin North Am 2008; 35: 81–89, vivi

[45] Zermann DH, Ishigooka M, Wunderlich H, Reichelt O, Schubert J. A study of pelvic floor function pre- and postradical prostatectomy using clinical neurourological investigations, urodynamics and electromyography. Eur Urol 2000; 37: 72–78

[46] Zermann DH, Ishigooka M, Doggweiler-Wiygul R, Schmidt RA. Chronic perineal pain and lower urinary tract dysfunction—a clinical feature of the "Gulf War syndrome"? World J Urol 2001; 19: 213–215

[47] Pontari M. Chronic prostatitis/chronic pelvic pain: the disease. J Urol 2009; 182: 19–20

[48] Zondervan KT, Yudkin PL, Vessey MP et al. Chronic pelvic pain in the community—symptoms, investigations, and diagnoses. Am J Obstet Gynecol 2001; 184: 1149–1155

[49] Zondervan KT, Yudkin PL, Vessey MP et al. The community prevalence of chronic pelvic pain in women and associated illness behaviour. Br J Gen Pract 2001b; 51: 541–547

[50] Martin-Alguacil N, Pfaff DW, Shelley DN, Schober JM. Clitoral sexual arousal: an immunocytochemical and innervation study of the clitoris. BJU Int 2008; 101: 1407–1413

[51] Giamberardino MA. Recent and forgotten aspects of visceral pain. Eur J Pain 1999; 3: 77–92

[52] Meeus M, Nijs J. Central sensitization: a biopsychosocial explanation for chronic widespread pain in patients with fibromyalgia and chronic fatigue syndrome. Clin Rheumatol 2007; 26: 465–473

[53] Tattersall JE, Cervero F, Lumb BM. Effects of reversible spinalization on the visceral input to viscerosomatic neurons in the lower thoracic spinal cord of the cat. J Neurophysiol 1986; 56: 785–796

[54] Ceravolo R, Nuti A, Siciliano G, Calabrese R, Bonuccelli U, Cellai F. A case of pelvic floor myoclonic jerk syndrome. Mov Disord 1996; 11: 331–333

[55] Cervero F, Laird JM. Understanding the signaling and transmission of visceral nociceptive events. J Neurobiol 2004; 61: 45–54

[56] Li J, Micevych P, McDonald J, Rapkin A, Chaban V. Inflammation in the uterus induces phosphorylated extracellular signal-regulated kinase and substance P immunoreactivity in dorsal root ganglia neurons innervating both uterus and colon in rats. J Neurosci Res 2008; 86: 2746–2752

[57] Berkley KJ, Hubscher CH, Wall PD. Neuronal responses to stimulation of the cervix, uterus, colon, and skin in the rat spinal cord. J Neurophysiol 1993; 69: 545–556

[58] Berkley KJ. A life of pelvic pain. Physiol Behav 2005; 86: 272–280

[59] Carter JE. Diagnosis and treatment of the causes of chronic pelvic pain. J Am Assoc Gynecol Laparosc 1996; 3 Supplement: S5–S6

[60] Carter JE. A systematic history for the patient with chronic pelvic pain. JSLS 1999; 3: 245–252

[61] Davila GW. Vaginal prolapse: management with nonsurgical techniques. Postgrad Med 1996; 99: 171–176, 181, 184–185

[62] Davila GW, Ghoniem GM, Kapoor DS, Contreras-Ortiz O. Pelvic floor dysfunction management practice patterns: a survey of members of the International Urogynecological Association. Int Urogynecol J Pelvic Floor Dysfunct 2002; 13: 319–325

[63] Davila GW, Guerette N. Current treatment options for female urinary incontinence—a review. Int J Fertil Womens Med 2004; 49: 102–112

[64] Chen MA, Davidson TM. Scar management: prevention and treatment strategies. Curr Opin Otolaryngol Head Neck Surg 2005; 13: 242–247

[65] Chen SY, Lin FS, Shen KH, Chen KC, Xiang P. [Non-invasive therapeutics in female urinary incontinence by extracorporeal magnetic innervation (ExMI)] Hu Li Za Zhi 2005; 52: 53–58

[66] Tympanidis P, Terenghi G, Dowd P. Increased innervation of the vulval vestibule in patients with vulvodynia. Br J Dermatol 2003; 148: 1021–1027

[67] Vander AJ, Sherman JH, Luciano DS, Eds. (1990). Human physiology. New York, St. Louis, San Francisco, Aukland, Bogota, Caracas, Hamburg, Lisbon, London, Madrid, Mexico, Milan, Montreal, New Delhi, Oklahoma City, Paris, San Juan Sao Paulo, Singapore, Sydney, Tokyo, Toronto: McGraw-Hill

[68] Anderson RU, Sawyer T, Wise D, Morey A, Nathanson BH. Painful myofascial trigger points and pain sites in men with chronic prostatitis/chronic pelvic pain syndrome. J Urol 2009; 182: 2753–2758

[69] Riedl A, Schmidtmann M, Stengel A et al. Somatic comorbidities of irritable bowel syndrome: a systematic analysis. J Psychosom Res 2008; 64: 573–582

[70] Khan KM, Cook JL, Maffulli N, Kannus P. Where is the pain coming from in tendinopathy? It may be biochemical, not only structural, in origin. Br J Sports Med 2000; 34: 81–83

[71] Khan KM, Cook JL, Taunton JE, Bonar F. Overuse tendinosis, not tendinitis part 1: a new paradigm for a difficult clinical problem. Phys Sportsmed 2000; 28: 38–48

[72] Aström M, Rausing A. Chronic Achilles tendinopathy. A survey of surgical and histopathologic findings. Clin Orthop Relat Res 1995: 151–164

[73] Cook JL, Khan KM, Maffulli N, Purdam C. Overuse tendinosis, not tendinitis part 2: applying the new approach to patellar tendinopathy. Phys Sportsmed 2000; 28: 31–46

[74] Leadbetter WB. Cell-matrix response in tendon injury. Clin Sports Med 1992; 11: 533–578

[75] Maffulli N, Wong J, Almekinders LC. Types and epidemiology of tendinopathy. Clin Sports Med 2003; 22: 675–692

[76] Phillips SM, Glover EI, Rennie MJ. Alterations of protein turnover underlying disuse atrophy in human skeletal muscle. J Appl Physiol (1985) 2009; 107: 645–654

[77] McPartland JM. Travell trigger points—molecular and osteopathic perspectives. J Am Osteopath Assoc 2004; 104: 244–249

[78] Travell JG, Simons DG, Lois LS, Eds. (1999). Myofascial pain & dysfunction: The trigger point manual. Philadelphia, Baltimore, New York, London, Buenos Aires, Hong Kong, Sydney, Tokyo: Lippincott Williams & Wilkins

[79] So C. How manipulation works. The Journal of the Hong Kong Physiotherapy Association, 1986; 8: 30-34

[80] Wilhelmi, BJ. Widened and hypertrophic scar healing treatment and management. Medscape 2013; http://emedicine.medscape.com/article/1298541-treatment. Accessed June 12, 2015

[81] Lehto M, Järvinen M. Collagen and glycosaminoglycan synthesis of injured gastrocnemius muscle in rat. Eur Surg Res 1985; 17: 179–185

[82] Lehto M, Duance VC, Restall D. Collagen and fibronectin in a healing skeletal muscle injury. An immunohistological study of the effects of physical activity on the repair of injured gastrocnemius muscle in the rat. J Bone Joint Surg Br 1985; 67: 820–828

[83] Maffulli N, Ewen SW, Waterston SW, Reaper J, Barrass V. Tenocytes from ruptured and tendinopathic achilles tendons produce greater quantities of type III collagen than tenocytes from normal achilles tendons. An in vitro model of human tendon healing. Am J Sports Med 2000; 28: 499–505

[84] Thompson JF, Roberts CL, Currie M, Ellwood DA. Prevalence and persistence of health problems after childbirth: associations with parity and method of birth. Birth 2002; 29: 83–94

[85] Atiyeh BS. Nonsurgical management of hypertrophic scars: evidence-based therapies, standard practices, and emerging methods. Aesthetic Plast Surg 2007; 31: 468–492, discussion 493–494

[86] Edwards J. (2003). Scar management. Nursing Standard (Royal College of Nursing (Great Britain): 1987), 17(52), 39–42

[87] Fujiwara T, Togashi K, Yamaoka T et al. Kinematics of the uterus: cine mode MR imaging. Radiographics 2004; 24: e19

[88] Stark M, Hoyme UB, Stubert B, Kieback D, di Renzo GC. Post-cesarean adhesions—are they a unique entity? J Matern Fetal Neonatal Med 2008; 21: 513–516

[89] Kuremu RT, Jumbi G. Adhesive intestinal obstruction. East Afr Med J 2006; 83: 333–336

[90] Mogren IM. Does caesarean section negatively influence the post-partum prognosis of low back pain and pelvic pain during pregnancy? Eur Spine J 2007; 16: 115–121

[91] Peters AA, Van den Tillaart SA. The difficult patient in gastroenterology: chronic pelvic pain, adhesions, and sub occlusive episodes. Best Pract Res Clin Gastroenterol 2007; 21: 445–463

[92] Drew MK, Sibbritt D, Chiarelli P. No association between previous Caesarean-section delivery and back pain in mid-aged Australian women: an observational study. Aust J Physiother 2008; 54: 269–272

[93] Alton TB, Gee AO. Classifications in brief: Young and Burgess classification of pelvic ring injuries. Clin Orthop Relat Res 2014; 8: 2338–2342

3 Evaluation

"The specific pathology underlying a patient's symptoms will dictate which treatment is most appropriate. Take, for example, the patient suffering from retrosternal chest pain of cardiac origin. These pains may mimic those of a patient suffering from thoracic spine pathology. While the subjective reports may be similar in nature, the treatments will be unique between the two pathologies.[1,2,3]

Learning Objectives

- The clinician will explain the appropriateness of evaluating the thoracic, lumbar, and sacral spines when working with the patient suffering with a pelvic pain.
- The clinician will demonstrate an evaluation of the patient with a pelvic pain.
- The clinician will formulate a functional diagnosis for the patient suffering with a pelvic pain based upon the findings from the evaluation.
- The clinician will make the determination as to when an internal pelvic examination is appropriate.

Due to the multitude of contributing neurological and segmental factors involved with the urogenital and visceral systems, the evaluation of the patient with pelvic pain is to be inclusive of the thoracic, lumbar, and sacral spines, and the sacroiliac joint (SIJ) and the coxofemoral joint. Serious pathology does exist, and must be considered when evaluating all patients; a differential diagnostic perspective must be maintained throughout the evaluation.

The thoracic spine is described as having the "capacity for much mischief,"[4] and the lumbar spine can refer pain and muscle spasm to the pelvic structures. Musculoskeletal disorders of the thoracic spine often mimic gastrointestinal, pulmonary, and cardiac conditions, whereas the viscera itself can produce symptoms that appear to be musculoskeletal.[4] When evaluating the patient with pelvic pain, despite contradictions in the orthopedic literature, the testing of the SIJ is considered necessary, as in a study by Lukban et al 100% of the subjects tested positive for SIJ dysfunction, and 94% reported an improvement of their dyspareunia after treatment, whereas diagnostic ultrasound (DUS) confirmed that patients with severe pregnancy-related pain had an asymmetrical laxity of the SIJ during pregnancy and demonstrated a threefold risk of moderate to severe postpartum pelvic pain.[5]

To date there is no gold standard for the evaluation of pelvic floor pain. A commonly accepted algorithm includes the collection of historical features such as deep pelvic pain, localized pelvic pain, dyspareunia, postcoital pain that lingers, with a physical examination that may include the saddle region inclusive of the pelvic floor musculature (PFM).

Unlike the evaluation of the axial structures where isolated testing is feasible, assessing the patient with pelvic pain requires greater interpretation and extrapolation. The clinician should have a concrete understanding of the visceral and osteokinematic anatomy, referral patterns of the various structures as they relate to the pelvis and perineum, as well as a functional understanding of the psychology of pain. Pelvic pain patients will often have a multitude of symptoms that are seemingly unrelated, but diagnostically invaluable. Deducing those symptoms that initiate and perpetuate the pain experience from those that are parallel in nature will assist in determining which treatment is most appropriate for each patient.

During the course of the evaluation the clinician can utilize the flowchart shown in ▶ Fig. 3.1, where Joint A, B, and C (noted as: Jt. A, Jt. B, Jt. C) are respective joints that the clinician will either rule in or rule out.

To avoid a hasty judgment or overlooking nongynecological causes of chronic pelvic pain, Carter et al recommend utilizing the acronym, GGUMPS to ensure a more accurate diagnosis.[6,7]

Gynecologic considerations:
- Endometriosis
- Adhesions (chronic pelvic inflammatory disease [PID])
- Leiomyoma
- Adenomyosis

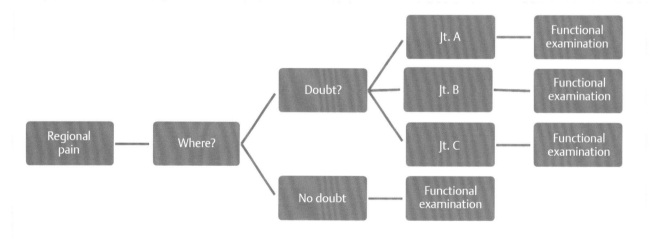

Fig. 3.1 Flowchart for conducting evaluation. Jt, joint.

- Pelvic congestion syndrome
- Mittelschmerz

Gastrointestinal considerations:
- Irritable bowel syndrome
- Chronic appendicitis
- Crohn's disease
- Inflammatory bowel disease
- Diverticulosis, diverticulitis
- Meckel's diverticulum

Urological considerations:
- Unstable bladder
- Detrusor instability
- Urethral syndrome
- Chronic urethritis
- Interstitial cystitis

Musculoskeletal/Neurological:
- Fibromyalgia
- Hernia
- Nerve entrapment
- Neuritis
- Fasciitis
- Scoliosis
- Disk disease
- Spondylolisthesis
- Osteitis pubis

Psychological considerations:
- Depression
- Anxiety
- Psychosexual dysfunction/abuse
- Hypochondriasis
- Somatization
- Personality disorder
- Cesarean section
- Episiotomy
- Adhesive disease
- Chronic appendicitis
- Hernia
- Inflammatory bowel disease

3.1 Initial Observation

The evaluation is to begin in the waiting room, as the patient is completing her intake paperwork. Observing the patient while she is acting independent of an actual "evaluation" will shed light on her sincerity and level of dysfunction. Caution is necessary when the observed behaviors in the waiting room vary drastically from those in the formal evaluating room. Movement patterns, postural proclivities, and gait anomalies are also to be documented while the patient is involved in activities that are not directly "evaluation" related: movement from car to office, filling out paperwork, and interacting with others while waiting for the evaluation to begin. Disparities give the clinician room for consideration when determining whether an internal evaluation is appropriate. Essentially, begin to deduce what is the general appearance and presentation of the patient, and whether behavior is consistent.

Summary of observations to make:
- Is she holding herself in a protected fashion?
- Is she interactive or withdrawn?
- Is she demonstrating distressed behaviors?
- Is she standing quietly or pacing the room?
- How does she move from the waiting room to the evaluation room?

3.2 History

Once the patient is in the evaluation room, a thorough history is to be taken. While conducting the verbal history, the clinician needs to listen for specific cues that will assist in ascertaining the patient's symptoms. The location and quality of symptoms should be elicited from the patient, who should be encouraged to be specific and concise. The purpose of subjective examination is to determine what the patient is experiencing, and how she relates to this experience. Using open-ended questions allows the patient to freely express herself, often offering information that is apropos to forming an accurate diagnosis. These questions allow the clinician the opportunity to evaluate the patient's perceived level of disability, her coping strategies, her support system, her emotional integrity, and to what degree her activities have been limited. The report of cramping pain is suggestive of visceral involvement, especially when it correlates with visceral dysfunction.[8,9,10,11,12,13] Visceral pain has been described as being a dull, poorly circumscribed ache that is experienced at various areas of the pelvis, whereas burning pain suggests neuropathic pain.[14]

Questions to be covered during the evaluation:
- Has she given birth?
  - Vaginally or cesarean section?
- Is she working?
  - What is required of her during vocational duties?
- Familial history of:
  - Endometriosis
  - Vulvar skin disease
- Does she have a sexually transmitted disease?
- When does she feel her pain?
  - What aggravates her pain?
  - What minimizes her pain?
- How does she cope with her pain?

Questions regarding child bearing, surgical history, and/or the presence of endometriosis are appropriate and necessary. Five to 20% of postpartum women experience pelvic girdle pain without a statistically significant difference between muscle thickness of the deep abdominal muscles and strength of their PFM.[15,16,17] It has been reported that second-stage labor places a 34.5% and 32.9% strain on the inferior and perineal nerve, respectively.[6,7] This is well beyond the 15 to 20% percent strain of a nerve that is known to cause nerve injury.[18,19,20]

It has been reported that 80% of the pelvic pain population[6,7] has endometriosis; this population is capable of localizing their pain to the site of the endometriosis lesion.[21]

Does the patient have a surgical history along the abdomen and/or saddle region that warrants further evaluation? Local scarring may impede mobility, strength of the underlying musculature, or be a source of low-level persistent pain.

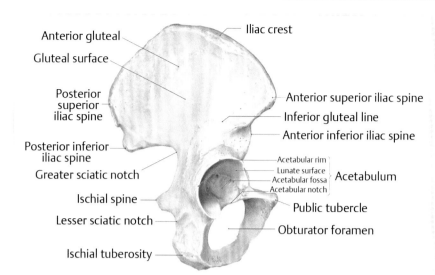

Anterior gluteal

Gluteal surface

Posterior superior iliac spine

Posterior inferior iliac spine

Greater sciatic notch

Ischial spine

Lesser sciatic notch

Ischial tuberosity

Iliac crest

Anterior superior iliac spine

Inferior gluteal line

Anterior inferior iliac spine

Acetabular rim
Lunate surface
Acetabular fossa   Acetabulum
Acetabular notch

Public tubercle

Obturator foramen

Fig. 3.2 Angle of declination. (From THIEME Atlas of Anatomy, General Anatomy and Musculo-skeletal System, © Thieme 2005, illustration by Karl Wesker.)

Clinical Note

It is often noted that a disassociation of the SIJ and the innominate is found when the patient has appropriate strength and function of the abdominals and a concurrent weakness of the pelvic floor.

The clinician's questions from this domain should include:

▶ **Do the symptoms indicate neurological entrapment?** Are the patient's symptoms referred? If so, what neurological structures can refer to the region outlined by the patient? Is there a specific dermatome outlined, or does the patient's pain indicate a cutaneous nerve entrapment? What joints, organs, and myofascial restrictions can refer to the region outlined by the patient? All must be considered while performing the evaluation.

Clinical Note

Appropriate treatment to the specific tissue at fault will provide improvements in the patients' wellness. These changes will be evident to both patient and clinician alike.

▶ **What influences the symptoms?**
▶ **How have the symptoms progressed or changed over time?**
After compiling this information, the clinician will begin to have an understanding as to why the patient has her symptoms, inclusive of an understanding of the various structures that may demonstrate these symptoms, and in this location. This suggests that every pain has a source, and it is the clinician's responsibility to determine the exact source to determine the appropriate treatment regimen.[3,22]

The last domain that the clinician will focus on is the extent to which the symptoms affect the patient's quality of life and how encompassing this problem is for this patient. How is this patient coping, and does she have the fortitude for an internal evaluation? During the course of the history taking, the clinician will be attempting to determine the patient's relative

state of anxiety associated with her pelvic pain condition, in addition to her general state of anxiety. There is a strong, positive correlation between anxiety, depression, and sexual dysfunction in women with chronic pelvic pain and the clinician must be cognizant of the patient's emotional maturity and disposition to minimize her risk to litigation and to ensure her comfort.[23,24]

During the medical history, the astute clinician will inquire about skin diseases elsewhere on the body, and also gather a family history of skin diseases as this patient may be more predisposed to developing vulvar skin diseases. The history should be inclusive of illnesses including diabetes mellitus, malignancy, and so forth.

3.3 Postural Observation and Inspection

The angle of declination is a measurement that is to be taken during the course of the evaluation, and it is defined as an imaginary line between the posterior superior iliac spine (PSIS) and the anterior superior iliac spine (ASIS), and is compared with the horizontal (▶ Fig. 3.2). A normative value for women is 10 to 20 degrees. An angle more than 20 degrees strongly indicates a weakness or inability to functionally utilize the abdominal and pelvic musculature. A lessening of the angle often leads to a flattening of the lumbar lordosis.

"Asymmetry is the norm," but it is also a component of soft-tissue changes of the paraspinal musculature, compensatory postures, and altered mechanics of the spine.[25] Al-Eisa et al found that those with either a lateral pelvic tilt (LPT), where the ASIS and PSIS was higher on one side, or an iliac rotation asymmetry (IRA),where the ASIS was higher and PSIS was lower, demonstrated significant differences in coupled lumbar rotation during lateral flexion than those with normal symmetry.[26,27] They concluded that subtle anatomic abnormalities of the pelvic bone alignment were associated with altered mechanics of the lumbar spine and that it may be a better indicator of functional deficit than absolute range of motion in individuals with lower back pain.[26,27] Therefore, when evaluating patients, noting positional asymmetries is appropriate to have a means of future comparison and also to assist in the formation of a functional diagnosis that is unique to each patient.

Clinical Note

Notice how the patient is holding their body.
   Teach them the most efficient means to hold themselves in order to reduce their pain, and promote healing.

Asymmetrical proclivities and postural habits can facilitate a series of muscle imbalances that will promote the shortening and tightening of muscle groups with antagonists elongating, demonstrating weaknesses and relative hypertrophy; atrophy of antagonistic musculature, along with a loss of fine motor control reflect a degradation of integrated muscle function.[25] Clinically, this is seen as the patient's way in which they hold themselves; in standing and in sitting. Muscles continually adapt to the body's orientation and postures as related to gravity; and faulty postures will result in an alteration of the center of gravity that will have consequences within the joints and muscular systems. Persistent aberrant afferent mechano-receptor facilitation due to faulty postures and positions will cause a change in spinal cord stimulation leading to muscle imbalances. Muscle balance will be altered in response to noxious stimuli and central mediation through the lateral reticular system, altering the activity of the gamma motor neurons, resulting in hyperreflexia and altered activation sequencing of muscle action; constant abhorrent neurological stimulation will increase the patient's experience of pain. This enhanced nociception will further facilitate alpha motor neurons segmentally, possibly leading to a progression of pain to a somatic structure that shares a common embryogenesis. Psychological predispositions can further influence muscle balance and resting tone.[25]

Clinical Note

Pain thresholds decrease and patient's pain increases when a noxious stimuli is applied for ≥ three-second intervals.

Often it is the case that the patient, in an attempt to stabilize the lumbosacral spine, is compliant with performing an abdominal strengthening regimen. If the pelvic floor musculature is compromised in any fashion, it is possible that a disassociation will occur between the innominate and the sacrum itself. In such a scenario the angle of declination may be appropriate while the sacrum is found to be hyper-nutated. The result is often palpable as globular nodules along the SIJ posteriorly. This is demonstrated in ▶ Fig. 3.3. The clinician should consider what has occurred to the anterior SIJ ligament in this scenario.

Clinical Note

The anterior SIJ ligament is often the cause of persistent SIJ pain and dysfunction and responds very well to local treatment.

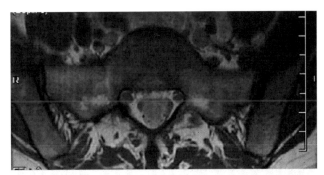
Fig. 3.3 Sacroiliac joint (SIJ), posteriorly.

3.4 Evaluation General Concepts

The clinician should incorporate a progressive schema when examining a patient with pelvic pain. This approach takes into consideration that the practitioner is accomplished at performing an evaluation and interpretation of the thoracic, lumbar, and sacral spines, as well as the hips and pelvic ring complexes. The proceeding framework is progressive in nature and allows the slow integration of the patient into the differential diagnostic model. This premise also helps the clinician decide whether or not it is appropriate to expose the saddle region and perform an internal examination. Evaluations must include a thorough medical history, a complete inspection, and a carefully conducted functional examination with any appropriate accessory tests. Upon completion of the evaluation, the clinician needs to interpret the resultant positive and negative findings that will offer insight into the origin of the pain and provide the basis of the clinical diagnosis.[3,22]

Despite the fact that the following framework is a symptom reproduction model, during the course of evaluating and treating a patient with pelvic pain the clinician will best serve the patient by having her avoid those activities and treatments that induce excessive pain or discomfort. The extent of a patient's experienced pain has a direct relationship between the number of painful experiences and the extent of hyperalgesia that patient experiences. The clinician, therefore, is to minimize painful experiences during the evaluation and subsequent treatment sessions.[8,9,10,11,12,13,28,29,30,31,32]

The clinician is to take into consideration that a woman's pain threshold fluctuates throughout her menstrual cycle. The tolerance to pain is less during the premenstrual phase and greatest during the luteal phase. Those suffering from dysmenorrhea will experience a greater reduction in their tolerance to pain after the cessation of their menses, especially along the abdomen.[30]

Finally, the clinician must be aware of the signs and symptoms of vulvar skin disease (▶ Fig. 3.4). Such signs and symptoms include: pruritus, burning, pain, soreness, changes in appearance of the vulva, or abnormal discharge. These patients will often complain about symptom exacerbation with micturition, intercourse, and the menstrual cycle. Examination of the vulvar region and perianal region will further assist in determining the possibility of a vulvar skin disease. Splits and fissures should be noted and questioned as to their duration. There are four types of skin conditions about which the clinician should be aware: (1)

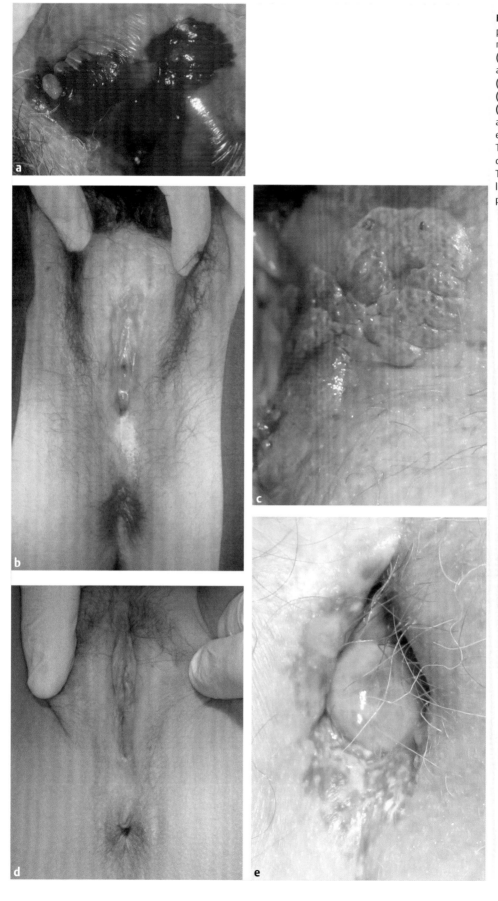

Fig. 3.4 a–e (a) Erythroplakia in a patient with high-grade squamous intraepithelial lesions. (b) Leukoplakia in a patient with advanced lichen sclerosus. (c) Squamous cell vulvar cancer. (d) Intermediate lichen sclerosus. (e) Psoriasis with silvery scaling and sharply demarcated erythema. (From Girardi F, Reich O, Tamussino K, Burghardt's Colposcopy and Cervical Pathology: Textbook and Atlas, Thieme Publishers, Stuttgart: 2014. Used with permission.)

inflammatory disorders, (2) infections, (3) tumors, and (4) blistering disorders. Inflammatory disorders include dermatitis (eczema), contact dermatitis, psoriasis, lichen planus, and lichen sclerosus. Infections include fungal, bacterial, viral, and infestations: candida, trichomonas vaginalis, and herpes. Tumors can be either benign or malignant, including malignant melanoma and squamous cell carcinoma. Blistering disorders include pemphigus and pemphigoid.[21,33,34,35,36]

During the course of the evaluation, the clinician will take note of specific movements and special tests (which will be discussed later in the text), to note how the patient responds. Do the actions and tests either produce or decrease the patient's symptom(s)? The clinician is to maintain a sound understanding of the various pain referral pattern of the involved anatomy and is to methodically rule each structure in or out as to whether or not it is causative in each patient's pain or dysfunction. Knowledge of common embryological origin of the visceral structures and their ability to refer intrasegmentally, within that segment to those somatic structures that share the same segment, is useful in making a diagnosis. Considering the multisegmental innervations of the viscera and PFM, the musculoskeletal screening portion of the examination includes the thoracic, lumbar, sacral spines, and the hip joints, noting subtle patterns to deduce a common segmental level of involvement or implication of a mechanical lesion of the spine or hip.[3,21,22,37] In summary, the clinician is to evaluate how the entire system is functioning as a whole. The following hierarchy is utilized in determining the likely pain-perpetuating source:

- Biopsychosocial factors
  - Somatization
  - Perseveration
  - Anxiety
- Neurological
  - Referred pain
  - Centralization, convergence, and sensitization
- Joint Restrictions
  - Facet inflammation/referred pain
  - Internal derangement of hip
  - Arthropathy
- Scar presence and restrictions
  - Abdominal
  - Perineal
  - Hip
- Muscle imbalance and generalized weakness
  - Postural faults
    - Sitting
    - Standing

Despite the contradictions in SIJ literature as related to the general orthopedic population, those patients with pelvic pain and a history of pregnancy tend to exhibit asymmetrical SIJ laxity. It has been found that subjects with moderate to severe pregnancy-related pain and asymmetrical laxity of the SIJ (as confirmed via DUS) have a threefold higher risk of moderate to severe postpartum pelvic pain.[38] One-hundred percent of the 16 subjects in the Lukban et al study tested positive for SIJ dysfunction with a 94% improvement of dyspareunia, painful sexual intercourse, after undergoing treatment directed at the SIJ.[5,39]

3.5 Spinal Examination

The evaluation of the patient suffering from pelvic pain and dysfunction is to be inclusive of the thoracic, lumbar, and sacral spines, in addition to the SIJs and the coxofemoral joints. Each of the aforementioned structures can refer pain to the pelvis, and must be ruled out prior to considering performing an internal evaluation. The examination process presented here follows the guidelines of Dr. James Cyriax. Unlike many orthopedic conditions where there are often many clinically definitive findings that implicate a particular structure as the source of the patient's pain, findings in the patient suffering with pelvic pain may not be as clear-cut. The clinician must take into consideration the aforementioned structures, their referral patterns, and the multitude of structures outlined previously when evaluating this patient population. The patient suffering from any chronic malady, let alone pelvic pain, will often have a plethora of ailments that lie over one another. This can be quite confounding to the novice and experienced clinician alike. During the course of the evaluation, the clinician is to note whether or not the findings of the evaluation are concurrent, causational, or correlational.[3,22,37]

> **Clinical Note**
>
> It is common that there be a visible decrease in osteokinematic motion at the segment(s) involved in a patient's pain.

Concurrent findings are those that parallel the patient's primary complaint. They may directly or indirectly perpetuate the patient's pain cycle. The most common example would be the attaining and maintaining of a forward flexed posture, a slouched position. In such a position, the dural tube is placed under considerable strain, and as was stated in the neurological discussion in Chapter 2, the dura mater is highly sensitive to stretch. This hyperkyphotic alignment of the spine also enhances the posterior migration of the intervertebral disks, further compromising dural mobility and increasing the likelihood of a disk lesion. Causational findings are those that test positive during the evaluation, where the symptoms are reproduced, and give a clear-cut diagnosis in this patient population. A common example would be the patient with an acute primary posterolateral disk lesion where a specific event initiated the patient's symptoms, and a specific movement reproduces these symptoms. Correlational findings will be the most nuanced and difficult to ascertain. The clinician will often have subtle hints as to the locality of pain origination and propagation. This is most commonly noted in the presence of a centrally sensitized segment of the spinal column. Often difficult to specifically test with one maneuver, the clinician is forced to make determinations based upon the composite of subtle indications and knowledge of the embryological derivation of the pelvic structures. ▶ Table 3.1 is a summary of the visceral structures and their embryological somites.

After having observed the patient's resting sitting and standing proclivities, and having noted the relative angle of declination, symmetry of stance, and ease to which they hold themselves (are they fidgeting?), the clinician can initiate the spinal screening. This begins with the patient standing with their back

Table 3.1 Visceral structures and their embryological somites

Organ/Joint	C3	C4	T6	T7	T8	T9	T10	T11	T12	L1	L2	L3	L4	L5	S1	S2	S3	S4	S5	Co1	Co2
Sternoclavicular joint	X	X																			
Pancreas				X	X																
Liver						X															
Gall Bladder			X	X	X	X	X														
Stomach/duodenum				X	X	X	X														
Small intestine						X	X														
Epididymis							X														
Colon: ascending							X	X	X	X											
Kidney							X	X	X	X											
Appendix							X	X	X	X											
Ureter								X	X	X											
Bladder fundus								X	X	X											
Uterine fundus								X	X	X											
Bladder Neck								X	X	X											
Vagina								X	X	X											
Suprarenal gland								X	X	X											
Ovary/testes								X	X	X											
Colon; flexure										X	X										
Colon; sigmoid											X	X									
Prostate																X	X	X	X		
Urethra																X	X	X	X		
Rectum																	X	X	X		

to the clinician. The clinician runs a hand down the length of the spine to note the presence of a step deformity, indicating the possible presence of a spondylolisthesis. After which time, the clinician rests his or her hands upon the iliac crest in full pronation with a firm, yet gentle pressure. This allows for the opportunity to notice the patient's tolerance to touch in addition to providing the clinician the means to determine whether or not there is symmetrical tone of the local musculature and relative iliac crest heights. While maintaining the pronated position of the forearm, the clinician is to sweep his or her thumbs along the posterior iliac crest in such a fashion that the subtle rise and fall can be appreciated. The sweeping thumb will rise, and then fall over the posterior aspect of the iliac crest posteriorly. Once the thumb has "fallen," the clinician is to turn the thumbs cranially, and then press up. There should be a feeling of a firm end. This is the PSIS; S2 can be found as a midpoint between the two PSISs. Next, the patient is asked to side bend to the left, and then right, and then to extend backward toward the clinician. Once those motions are completed, and with the clinician's palpating digits upon the PSIS, the patient is asked to forward flex. This is the standing flexion test of the SIJ. A greater migration of one of the PSIS points as compared with the opposite indicates that a hypomobility may exist on the side that moved the greatest. The following test, known as the Gillet test (or march test, or stork test) is then readily performed as the clinician's hands are prepositioned. With one palpating digit maintained at the PSIS, the opposite thumb is moved to the sacral body. The clinician then asks the patient to flex the hip that corresponds to the thumb that is maintained at the PSIS. During the movement of the hip, the clinician notes the relative movement of the PSIS thumb to that of the sacral thumb. Normal movement is considered when the PSIS thumb moves first and the sacral thumb moves second. Hypomobility of the ipsilateral SIJ is suspected when the two, PSIS and sacrum, move as a unit. These two findings together allow the clinician the opportunity to appreciate the local mobility of the SIJ, and its potential as a pain generator can be appreciated.

> **Clinical Note**
>
> The author respects the fact that current research questions the validity, and reliability of SIJ movement tests.
>
> The author, however, has found that when used in conjunction with accurate palpation they prove to be very useful in the formation of a functional diagnosis.

The patient is then asked to stand facing the clinician. The patient and clinician then lightly hold hands as the patient is asked to stand on one foot, and then to perform 10 heel raises; this is to assess the S1 nerve root. If the SIJ is suspect, a drop heel test can be performed by having the patient assume maximal unilateral plantarflexion and then to "drop" the calcaneous to the floor; pain at the SIJ is a positive test (▶ Fig. 3.5).

The evaluation is then taken to the sitting position, where the patient is taken into passive scapular approximation to assess the C8 to T2 nerve roots, and with cervical flexion; the dural mobility can be appreciated. If a thoracic lesion is suspected, both active and passive rotation can be evaluated at this time.

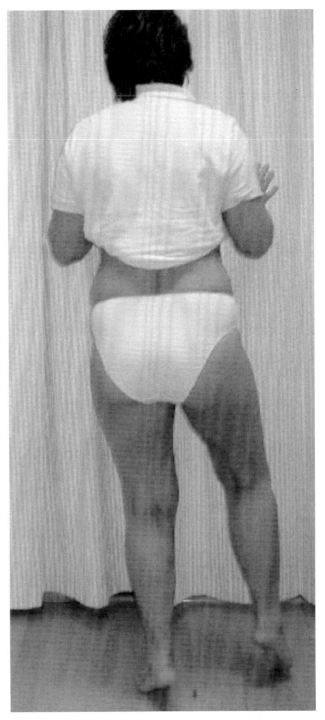

Fig. 3.5 Drop heel test.

The patient is then asked to assume the supine position. Either one or both of their forearms are placed at the lumbar lordosis to provide stability. With the patient supine, the clinician assesses the straight leg raise maneuver by slowly bringing the leg into hip flexion while maintaining the knee in terminal extension. If tensioning of the sciatic nerve is experienced by the patient commenting on pain, or if the clinician "feels" the sciatic nerve tension, the foot can be taken into dorsiflexion, and the cervical spine flexed according to the tests as described by Neri to further discriminate the mobility of the dura mater.[40]

Upon completion of the straight leg raising test, the clinician is in a good position to assess passive hip flexion by flexing the knee and approximating the patient's knee toward their chest. Then, by withdrawing to 90 degrees of hip flexion, both internal and external rotation can be assessed. If a labral lesion is suspected, the hip can be taken into maximal adduction and then internally rotated. With the patients' thigh being stabilized across the clinician's sternum, and counter pressure being applied to the patient's abdomen, the L2 nerve root/myotome can be inspected by having the patient actively flex their hip. The clinician can then assess the SIJ by performing the Östgaard test by taking his or her caudal hand and placing it under the patient's sacrum and, while maintaining the patient in 90 degrees of hip flexion, providing a shearing force through the SIJ by compressing the patient's knee to their sternum and driving force through the femur, with the axial pressure being held for one minute. A positive test is the production of local pain at the SIJ. The clinician then allows the patient to relax their legs to the table, as he or she remains in position over the patient's pelvis. The clinician places his or her palms along the lateral margin of the ASIS and applies a compressive force through the pelvis, compressing the pubic symphysis and distracting the SIJs. This is held for one minute. Positive tests are those that provoke pain. After one minute, the clinician assumes the cross-armed position while maintaining position over the patient's pelvis. The palms of the hand are placed along the medial border of the ASIS and a pressure is applied laterally, gapping the pubic symphysis and compressing the SIJs posteriorly.

To further assess the involvement of the SIJ and its ligaments, the following procedures can be employed:
- Iliolumbar ligament:
  ○ The patient's flexed hip is adducted toward the contralateral hip.
  ○ At maximal adduction, an axial pressure is applied through the femur.
  ○ A positive examination will be noted as the provocation of pain to the inguinal region; care is to be taken to rule out hip labral pathology to make this diagnosis.

- Sacrospinous and posterior sacroiliac ligaments:
  ○ The patient's flexed hip is adducted toward the contralateral shoulder.
  ○ At maximal adduction, an axial pressure is applied through the femur.
  ○ A positive examination will be the provocation of pain along the S1 dermatome.
- Sacrotubral ligaments:
  ○ The patient's hip is maximally flexed toward the ipsilateral shoulder.
  ○ At maximal hip flexion, an axial pressure is applied through the femur.
  ○ A positive examination will be the provocation of pain throughout the S1 dermatome.

The inspection of local scars is then to be performed, noting their location, pliability, and symptom provocation. The clinician is to have a consistent manner to which he or she approaches scars as to ensure consistency and repeatability. Starting superior and moving inferiorly or moving from the left-most margin to the right-most margin is a common strategy (► Fig. 3.6).[41] The clinician is to assess the pliability of the scar in the following fashion: A palpating digit is placed along the incision, often starting on a particular edge (left, for example). While maintaining strict skin-to-scar contact between the palpating digit and the scar, the scar is to be deflected in a leftward, then rightward, then upward, and then downward fashion. This is often described as if referencing a compass: east to west, north to south (► Fig. 3.7, ► Fig. 3.8, ► Fig. 3.9, and ► Fig. 3.10).

The clinician next slides his or her hand down the length of the patient's leg, stopping at the knee. While holding the knee in modest flexion (~30 degrees), the deep tendon reflex (DTR) of the patella can be assessed (L3).

Then, moving more caudally, the clinician assesses the lumbar dermatomes, or conduct light touch sensation discrimination bilaterally as previously outlined. The supine test then concludes with the assessment of the extensor Babinski reflex by stroking the reflex hammer along the sole of the patient's foot. Manual muscle testing (MMT) of the lumbar plexus can be performed at this point in time also as the clinician is at the patient's feet. With the patient supine the distal tibia can be

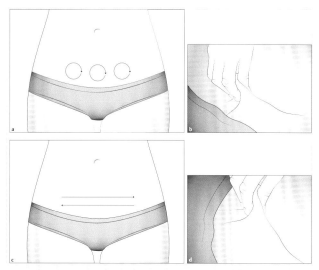

Fig. 3.6 a–d Scar management techniques.

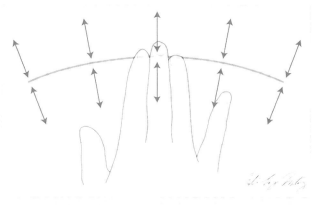

Fig. 3.7 From Wallace, K. Reviving Your Sex Life after Childbirth; your guide to pain-free and pleasurable sex after the baby. 2014. Used with permission.

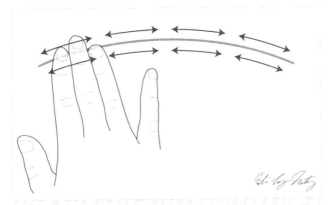

Fig. 3.8 From Wallace, K. Reviving Your Sex Life after Childbirth; your guide to pain-free and pleasurable sex after the baby. 2014. Used with permission.

patient's abdomen along the location of the pain, locating and provoking the pain through palpation, and then having the patient perform a partial sit-up. During the sit-up maneuver the patient's pain is assessed. A diminishing of the pain indicates the possible presence of visceral involvement, whereas an increase of local pain indicates the presence of a tendinopathy of the abdominal musculature. An additional observation that the clinician can make during the performance of the sit-up motion is known as the Beever's sign. During the sit-up motion, the clinician takes notice of the umbilicus. During a sit-up the umbilicus normally maintains one position; it doesn't move. If movement is seen, the clinician is to notice the direction of movement. Superior migration indicates a lesion along the T10–12 nerve root, superior and lateral migration indicates a T10–12 nerve root lesion opposite the side of movement, whereas an inferior migration indicates a T7–10 nerve root lesion, and an inferior and lateral migration indicates a T7–10 nerve root lesion opposite the side of movement. An additional observation to make during the performance of a sit-up is the presence of diastasis recti. The abdominal reflex can be performed at this time with the use of a pinwheel, or the end of a reflex hammer. This test is performed by stroking each quadrant of the abdomen toward the umbilicus. The umbilicus is to move toward the stroking instrument, and an absence indicates a possible lower motor nerve lesion at T7-L2. If a local tendinopathy is suspected of the hip adductors, testing should be performed at zero degrees of hip flexion, to rule out the Gracilis; at

stabilized with one hand, while the other hand (using the web space along the talus) provides a resistance point to dorsiflexion (L4). While stabilizing the tibia, the clinician's hand is moved laterally from the talus to the lateral aspect of digit five to resist eversion(L5-)S1. And finally, bilateral great toe extension is assessed (L4–5).

An additional series of tests can be performed. The first is to be included when visceral disease is suspected. This test is known as Carnett's test. It is performed by palpating the

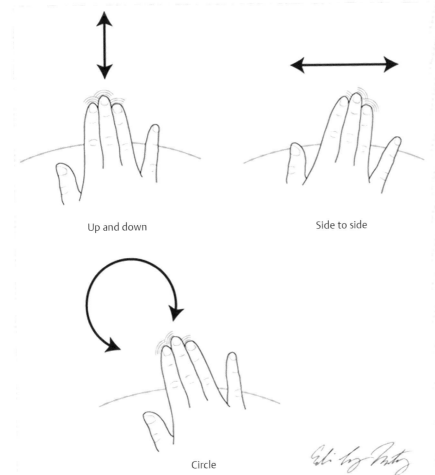

Fig. 3.9 From Wallace, K. Reviving Your Sex Life after Childbirth; your guide to pain-free and pleasurable sex after the baby. 2014. Used with permission.

Up and down

Side to side

Circle

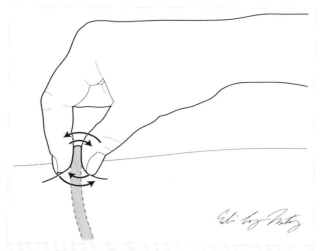

Fig. 3.10 From Wallace, K. Reviving Your Sex Life after Childbirth; your guide to pain-free and pleasurable sex after the baby. 2014. Used with permission.

feel a fasciculation under his or her palpating hand at L1–3. After performing the prone knee flexion maneuver, the clinician is to stabilize the distal femur, and resist both knee flexion and then extension: S1–2 and L3–4, respectively. Upon completion, the Achilles DTR assessment can be performed by placing the ankle into dorsiflexion. A pincer grip is then taken at the bilateral gluteus maximus. The patient is asked to contract the glutei together. A disparity of strength may indicate a lesion to the S2 nerve root, or SIJ inflammation ("dead butt" syndrome). The clinician is then to palpate for S2 as previously described. A sacral thrust is then performed by the clinician placing a hypothenar pressure, reinforced by a split finger/hand. The central posterior-to-anterior CPA is held for one minute and is used to assess relative mobility and symptom provocation. The clinician is then to continue the CPA through the lumbar spine, and into the thoracic spine if the clinician has reason to suspect involvement of the thoracolumbar segments. Each CPA is to be initiated as a "stretch assessment," during which time the clinician is to assess the patient's tolerance to arthrokinematic motion, determining whether or not the patient's presenting symptoms are altered: aggravated or reduced.

45 degrees of flexion, to rule out the adductor longus and pubic symphysis; and at 90 degrees of flexion, to rule out the pectineus.

With the patient in prone position, the examination continues with the passive knee flexion test to assess the mobility of the femoral nerve. Care is to be taken during the performance of this procedure, and a gently placed hand across the L1–3 segments will often provide information on the presence of appropriate neural mobility (▶ Fig. 3.11). When there is tethering of these nerves, during passive knee flexion the clinician will often

Clinical Note

L1-3 ZAJ refer to the posterior SIJ region and corresponding hip musculature and is often misinterpreted as "piriformis syndrome."

To assess the posterior labrum, with the patient in lying prone the clinician takes the hip into passive hyperextension and then

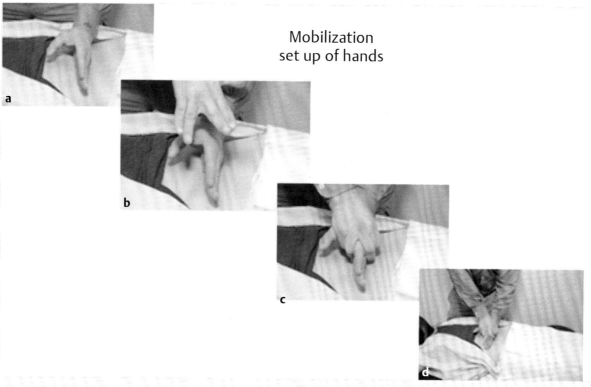

Mobilization
set up of hands

Fig. 3.11 a–d Mobilization: setup of hands.

maximal abduction, and then it is externally rotated. Pain provocation may indicate a tear of the posterior labrum.

3.6 Pelvic Examination—Concepts

Prior to performing a pelvic examination, the clinician is to take into consideration the findings to date. To maximize patient modesty, and provide optimal care, the clinician makes the determination whether or not the patient requires a pelvic examination. The following will assist the clinician in making this decision:

Is your patient able to sit? According to Nantes criterion, in true pudendal neuralgia the patient will be unable to sit, and the performance of an internal evaluation is appropriate to determine the location and reason for the pudendal neuralgia.[42]

Does the patient demonstrate asymmetrical proclivities in standing or sitting? Were there restrictions of the hip and or spinal segments, and were symptoms referred to the patient's pelvis? Did a mobilization to either the hip or spine influence the symptoms? If so, an internal evaluation can be deferred. If not, the performance of an internal evaluation would be appropriate. Were the evaluation tests and measures negative to date, and is the patient's presentation mature and sincere? If so, the performance of an internal evaluation would be appropriate so as to determine the cause of the pain.

Is there a history of trauma to the saddle region? Surgical? Birthing? Traumatic? If so, the performance of an internal evaluation may be appropriate.

During the course of the evaluation, were there any segmental restrictions of motion, or segmental losses of strength? Did that segment represent a segment that relates to the viscus embryogenetic origin? If so, did the provision of a mobilization to that segment influence the patient's symptoms and presenting findings? If so, an internal evaluation may be deferred. If not, an internal evaluation may be appropriate.

The purpose of the internal examination is to accurately assess the ability of the musculature of the pelvic floor to contract and relax voluntarily, to note the relative status of the muscle strength and bulk,[43,44,45,46,47,48,49] to note any scars or fibrotic lesions within the vaginal and rectal canal, and to attain a positional sense of the anatomy.[45,46,48] An accurate assessment of the PFM is functionally impossible via an external means, as it would necessitate assessing the musculature through the fat-filled ishiorectal fossa, which may be 10 cm thick.[50] Although digital palpation of pelvic floor defects assessment is poor when compared with three- and four-dimensional DUS,[43,44] it does provide a cost-effective strategy for a clinician to perform an evaluation. With practice and attention to details while performing an internal evaluation, a clinician can attain 70.2% accuracy in recognizing the internal pelvic structures.[51] Trained clinicians detected muscle defects in 9 of 29 women; expert clinicians detected muscle defects in 13 of 29 women.[51] Eight of 29 clinicians found the correlation between a lack of muscle bulk as a predictor of organ prolapse and stress urinary incontinence. It should be noted that they compared the palpable muscle "bulk" versus measuring strength or endurance.[52,53]

Levator ani muscle trauma is a common consequence of vaginal delivery and is detectable with digital vaginal palpation. Levator defects were found by Dietz and colleagues in 20% of subjects, with 81% agreement between assessors.[43,46,49]

Palpation detection of major levator trauma is less repeatable than identification by DUS.[43,46,49] Avulsion injury was diagnosed on palpation if there was a detachment of puborectalis muscle from its insertion on the inferior pubic ramus. Detection was via palpable bulging of muscle upon contraction. Consistent detection was found to occur in 80% of the cases where either the muscle is completely normal or completely avulsed. During the evaluation, difficulties exist with this method of evaluation while working with a patient who has relatively thin and atrophic musculature. Those with partial tears, denervation, or who demonstrate a generally low tone require a great deal of clinical competence in order to detect the lesion.[43,46,49]

> **Clinical Note**
>
> As the patient strengthens her pelvic floor, the local breaches in muscular integrity are often more prominent and more readily detected.

Avulsions of the puborectalis musculature may occur as a result of vaginal delivery and are associated with organ prolapse and with anal sphincter tearing, and resultant fecal incontinence, and also are related to maternal age at first delivery and the use of forceps during vaginal delivery.[44,49]

Prior to the visual inspection and physical performance of an internal examination, the patient must be offered appropriate education concerning what the evaluation entails and then provide/sign an informed consent document. The American Physical Therapy Association (APTA) states that internal examinations and treatments are well within the realm of physical therapists' skills sets and are appropriate in the evaluation and treatment of specific ailments. Although not required, it is suggested to have a third person present to minimize the risk to litigation. The recommendation by the APTA is inclusive of all internal physical therapy evaluations and treatments.[54]

Prior to initiating the pelvic examination, have the patient properly draped from the abdomen to the feet. Allow them to comfortably acquaint themselves to the concept of a pelvic examination, and confirm their comfort verbally. It is recommended that prior to visualizing the saddle region, let alone contacting the genitals, that the clinician obtain verbal permission from the patient. The clinician is to be as professionally clear in the request for permission to contact the pelvis, or the pelvic structures inclusive of the genitalia. Giving the patient control of what is going to be touched and when assists in alleviating anxiety, and ensures the patient that they are ultimately in control of who contacts their body, and where.

If it is necessary to perform a vaginal and rectal examination and treatment on the same visit, it is imperative that the clinician remove gloves after evaluating and treating one area and put on clean gloves prior to evaluating and treating the other. By doing so, the clinician will decrease the likelihood of involuntarily passing along human papillomavirus (HPV) and other contact viruses, diseases, and bodily fluids. HPV can remain viable for a week despite desiccation.[55]

External examination of the genitals and perineum[56] provides the clinician with information regarding the condition of the skin, perineal scars, and the trophic status of vaginal opening, otherwise known as the vaginal introitus, as well as regarding

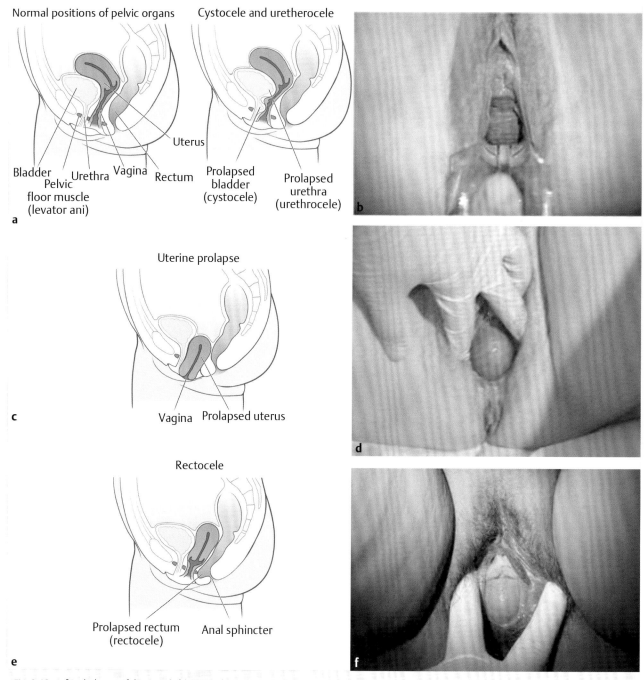

Fig. 3.12 a–f Pathologies of descent. **(a,b)** Cystocele. **(c,d)** Uretherocele. **(e,f)** Rectocele. (From Reece, EA, Barbieri, RL, Obstetrics and Gynecology: The Essentials of Clinical Care, Thieme Publishers, Stuttgart: 2010. Used with permission.)

the relationship between the posterior commissure and the external urethral meatus, elevation of the perineum, and signs of descent at rest (▶ Fig. 3.12).

The anterior vaginal wall should be found to be above the hymenal ring.[21] Descent is characteristic of an urethrocele and may be caused by one of three things:

1. Separation of the paravaginal attachment of the pubovesical fascia
2. Loss of the vagina's attachment to the cervix
3. Tearing of the pubovesical fascia with resultant herniation of the bladder, cystocele

If the cervix is found to be within 1 cm of the hymenal ring, a considerable loss of support is confirmed, a uterine prolapse. A defect in the rectovaginal fascia will be noted as a posterior migration of the vagina below the hymenal ring. Rectoceles and posterior enteroceles exist when the cul de sac becomes distended with the intestine and bulges the posterior vaginal wall.

During the initial observation of the saddle region and genitalia, the clinician is to take note of the resting tone of the pelvis to glean an appreciation for the patient's status. Is the perineum elevated and does there appear to be increased resting tone? If so, the clinician is to proceed with caution as the patient may be suffering from an ailment that renders the pelvic floor hypertonic. Are there signs of pelvic relaxation? Such signs may be labial separation and possible leakage of urine.

During the course of the evaluation, the clinician with a thorough understanding of anatomy will discern the presence of a tendinopathy often through palpation and MMT. This understanding and appreciation of the pelvic musculature is imperative so that the clinician can be as accurate as possible when discerning the PFM. MMT may require pre-tensioning of the desired muscle for the patient to sense whether or not the patient is able to contract the muscle, and whether or not the contraction provokes pain. This is easily accomplished with the musculature having coxofemoral joint attachments. For those muscles that do not have a coxofemoral attachment, a pre-tension can be applied by manually tensioning the muscle in a fashion that is parallel to the fiber orientation, away from the bony attachment.[57,58,59,60] Palpable for crepitation and swelling are common for the acute tendinopathy, with associated edema and hyperemia within the paratenon. The more chronic tendinopathy will present with lesser crepitations and edema than that of the acute lesion, but with an exaggeration of the paratendon thickening due to the fibrinous exudates and proliferation of myofibroblasts, and adhesions.[57,58,59,60] Discriminatory palpation by theclinician will find crepitus to be present in those tissues that are adversely affected. The crepitus will be noted as a granular sensation under the palpating digit, and is often accompanied by tenderness and pain.[57,59]

The MMT will also give the clinician information on the ability of the musculature to initiate a contraction. That which is strong but painful indicates a local musculotendionous lesion. Whereas a contraction that is weak and painful indicates an acute avulsion injury or a larger more acute musculotendinous injury. When an MMT is weak and painless it indicates a greater breach of the musculotendinous structure (grade III), or a compromise of neurological integrity. As would be performed when evaluating the peripheral joints, where the clinician would evaluate and compare the right versus the left when determining the degree to which the involved structure is compromised, the use of a split finger technique is a means to determine whether or not there is an asymmetry of the PFM (▶ Fig. 3.13). This split finger technique is to be conducted at each layer of the pelvic floor, and the results comparing the left to the right, from layer one, two, and three, are to be noted.

Prior to performing a pelvic examination, the clinician is to take into consideration their findings to date. In order to maximize patient modesty, and provide optimal care, the clinician is to make the determination whether or not their patient requires a pelvic examination. The following will assist the clinician in making this decision:

Is your patient able to sit? According to Nante's Criterion, in true pudendal neuralgia the patient will be unable to sit, and the performance of an internal evaluation is appropriate to determine the location and reason for the pudendal neuralgia.

Does the patient demonstrate asymmetrical proclivities in standing or sitting? Were there restrictions of the hip and or spinal segments, and were symptoms referred to the patient's pelvis? Did a mobilization to either the hip or spine influence the symptoms? If so, an internal evaluation may be deferred. If not, the performance of an internal evaluation would be appropriate. Was the evaluation negative to date, and the patient

presents as mature and sincere? If so, the performance of an internal evaluation would be appropriate so as to determine the cause of their pain.

Is there a history of trauma to the saddle region? Surgical? Birthing? Traumatic? If so, the performance of an internal evaluation may be appropriate.

During the course of the spinal screening and evaluation, were there any segmental restrictions of motion, or segmental losses of strength? Did that or those spinal segment(s) reflect a region of the spine whose somatic structure is representative of the patient's symptoms from an embryological perspective? If so, did the provision of a mobilization to that segment influence the patient's symptoms and presenting findings? If so, an internal evaluation may be deferred. If not, an internal evaluation may be appropriate.

> **Clinical Note**
>
> There is often an association between ipsilateral SIJ dysfunction and a decreased bulbospongiosus reflex, and a weakened but pain-free manual muscle testing of the pelvic musculature.

3.7 Pelvic Examination: The Performance

To maximize patient modesty, a gown or draping sheet is to be placed over the patient covering the abdomen to the feet. The clinician is to sit aside the plinth. With the patient resting comfortably in the lithotomy position (supine with hips/knees flexed), the clinician will request permission to observe the genital region (▶ Fig. 3.14). Once obtained, the examination will then initiate with a visual inspection of the saddle region. The clinician is to observe whether or not there are signs and symptoms of vulval skin disease. What is the condition of the external anatomy of the genitalia and anal region? Are there signs of scars? What is the trophic status of the vaginal introitus? Are there any signs of descent as noted by a physical presence exiting the vagina, or asymmetrical closure of the labia? Is there any leakage originating from the vagina or anus? Is the perineum held in an elevated or depressed position?

After the observation, the examination is to proceed by asking the patient to contract the PFM. The labia are to be observed and monitored. The perineal structures, such as the clitoris, are expected to demonstrate a posterior displacement, with a narrowing and inward movement of the introitus, shortening and drawing in of the perineum, and a retraction of the anus. A synergistic contraction of the abdominals, glutei, and/or adductors is to be noted as inappropriate, and verbal cues are to be given to allow the patient to isolate the PFM. The patient is then asked to cough. The clinician should note a reflexive contraction of the PFM (assessing the integration of T6 to L1 and S4–5), while taking note of any leakage or decent (may be seen as labial separation), opening of the introitus, gapping of the vagina, descent of the perineum, and/or prolapsing of the vaginal wall.

A gentle approach is to be taken when initiating contact with the perineum. The patient may be exquisitely tender, anxious, or both. Obtaining permission while stating what you are proposing

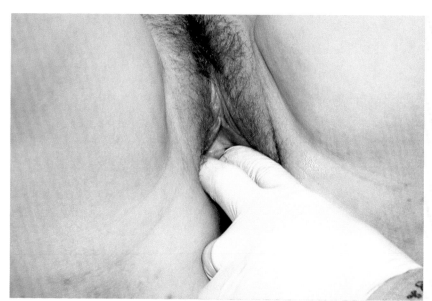

Fig. 3.13 Split-finger manual muscle test.

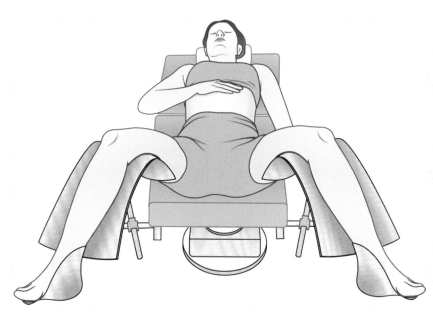

Fig. 3.14 Lithotomy position. (From Reece, EA, Barbieri, RL, Obstetrics and Gynecology: The Essentials of Clinical Care, Thieme Publishers, Stuttgart: 2010. Used with permission.)

to inspect will often alleviate any heightened anxiety and promote greater patient control of her physical wellness. With the clinician sitting aside the plinth, the patient resting comfortably in the lithotomy position, the clinician is to initiate contact along the adductor origin to the proximal pubis, a region that is minimally intimate, at approximately 9:00 on the perineal "clock.'"

Palpation of the saddle region is to proceed in a systematic fashion as outlined below. The purpose of proceeding in the outlined fashion is that it is a nonthreatening means to assess the patient's tolerance to contact, and to evaluate the first layer of pelvic musculature and structures. Due to the abundance of noncontractile tissue, a gentle contraction of the PFM can be used to confirm whether or not the clinician is in fact palpating a muscle or local noncontractile tissue.

Following the map in ▶ Fig. 3.15, the palpation process begins at the ischial tuberosity with a firm, yet progressive pressure.

At the ischial tuberosity the external transverse perineal musculature originates and the clinician can assess for continuity, crepitus, tenderness, and tone. The evaluation will continue with a palpating index finger gently pressing anteriorly and slightly superiorly toward the clitoris. As this digit progresses, it will assess the ischiocavernosus for continuity, crepitus, tenderness, and tone. Prior to reaching the clitoris, the clinician will deflect the clitoral hood as the patient may suffer from scarring that impedes its mobility and that may be a pain generator for the patient. Once appropriate clitoral hood mobility is noted, a gentle palpation with a pincer grip can be used to assess the bulbospongiosus continuity, crepitus, tenderness, and tone. At the perineum, the clinician is to re-direct the palpating digit toward the ischial tuberosity from where the assessment was begun of the insertion and body of the superficial transverse perineal muscle for continuity, crepitus, tenderness, and tone. A

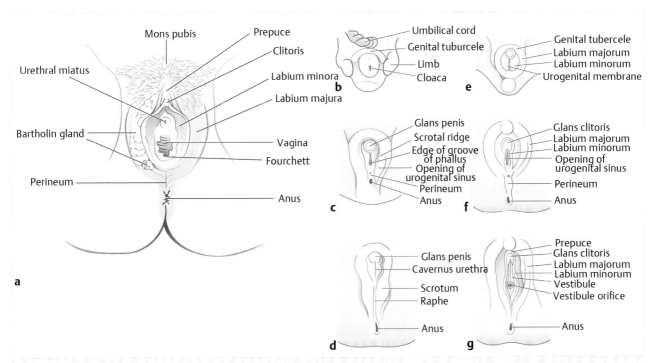

Fig. 3.15 a-g Vaginal palpation map. (From Reece, EA, Barbieri, RL, Obstetrics and Gynecology: The Essentials of Clinical Care, Thieme Publishers, Stuttgart: 2010. Used with permission.)

similar technique is to be employed for the male patient, with the obvious exception of the clitoral hood deflection. Deflection of the shaft of the penis may provide information, but is less likely to be a pain generator then it would be for the female clitoral hood.

At this time the labia minora, the smaller, thinner skin folds of the vagina, can be inspected for color continuity, presence of lesions, and general tissue mobility; adhesions may be a pain generator. Running of the finger and thumb in opposition throughout the length of the labia minora should be not result in pain, and the labia minora should be pliable. The integrity of the vulvar vestibule is to be discerned with the clinician inspecting the integrity of the posterior fourchette, hymenal remnants, vestibular glands, Skene's glands, and urethra. The Hart's line is the line that separates the labia minora from the vestibule and should be comfortably pliable to palpation. During the inspection process, in addition to noting pain provocation and muscle/fascial pliability, the clinician is to note a continuity of coloration, symptoms of inflammation, warts, bumps, and sores.

The examination continues with an assessment of the PFM (▶ Fig. 3.16). It is advised that the musculature be evaluated from layer one, two, and then three, and a comparison between the right and the left are to be made and documented. Just as with a shoulder affliction, the pelvic musculature can experience a dysfunction and injury unilaterally, and it is up to the clinician to determine whether or not there are asymmetrical findings when testing the function of the pelvic floor. The clinician evaluates for overall strength of the musculature, endurance of the musculature as noted in total hold time and number of single "quick" contractions the patient can make prior to fatiguing. A split finger technique can also be utilized to assess the

patient's ability to coordinate the two sides, and relative strength and endurance as noted above, layer to layer. This technique is helpful when gross asymmetries were not noted, or were difficult to assess. Where asymmetries present themselves, it is up to the clinician to determine the reason for these findings. Is there a local scar? Are there findings of neural entrapment? Is the anterior SIJ ligament inflamed and reflexively inhibiting local muscle activity?

Clinical Note

It is common to find SIJ hypomobility, a hyporeactive bulbospongiousus reflex, and unilateral weakness of the PFM.

After performing the layer three MMT the clinician will have full digital penetration into the vagina. A vaginal sweep is then performed to assess for tissue continuity (▶ Fig. 3.17). Using a sweeping motion with the palpating digit along both sidewalls will provide the clinician with information regarding local tissue continuity, crepitus, tenderness, and tone. Care must be taken to appreciate the individual patient's rugae, or natural vaginal contours and texture. It is common for the suffering patient to exclaim, "That is it!" when the taut scar band is initially palpated. Tenderness and muscle nodules are to be evaluated throughout the 360 degrees of the vaginal canal.

After performing the vaginal sweep, palpation of S2 can be done by further introduction of the palpating digit into the vagina in a posterior superior fashion, using the posterior inferior aspect of the pubic symphysis as a guide until the anterior aspect of the sacrum is encountered (▶ Fig. 3.18).

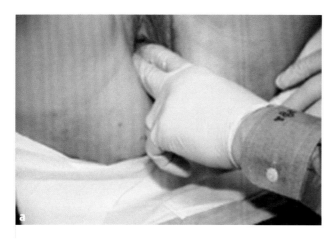

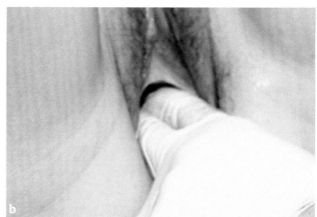

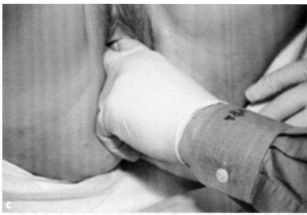

Fig. 3.16 a–c Split finger assessment of the pelvic floor musculature: layers one, two, and three.

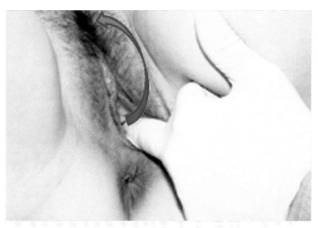

Fig. 3.17 Vaginal sweep.

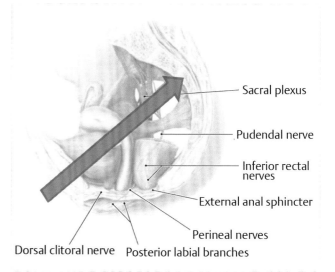

Sacral plexus

Pudendal nerve

Inferior rectal nerves

External anal sphincter

Perineal nerves

Dorsal clitoral nerve   Posterior labial branches

Fig. 3.18 Palpation of S2. (From THIEME Atlas of Anatomy, General Anatomy and Musculoskeletal System, © Thieme 2005, illustration by Karl Wesker.)

After having palpated for S2, the clinician slides this palpating digit laterally, toward him/herself, noting the anterior sacral sulci. A Tinel test can then be performed along the anterior aspect of the sacrum, comparing right to left and noting whether or not symptom reproduction is found. From the pal-

pation of sacral nerves 1 to 4, the clinician will move further laterally where the digit will feel as if it "falls off a cliff" only to find itself abutting into another firm structure, the ischial spine. From there, the clinician carefully palpates Alcock's canal, where again a Tinel test can be performed. The obturator internus may also be palpated at this time by directing the palpating digit in a superior lateral fashion, feeling akin to a "trampoline" that firms with hip abduction MMT.

Finally, the performance of the bulbospongiosus reflex is tested by taking the first digit of the clinician's palpating hand, and flexing it to 90 degrees and resting it along the lateral aspect of the clitoral hood (or in the male the base of the penis) (▶ Fig. 3.19). The internal digit is to remain (for extra sensitivity to testing procedure), and the fifth digit is to press firmly but gently at the external anal sphincter. A DTR hammer is then applied to the clinician's interphalangeal joint with extraordi-

nary care not to strike the patient. A rapid contraction of the PFM and/or external anal sphincter is appropriate. Asymmetries are to be noted and addressed. This procedure assesses the afferent limb of the clitoral branch of the pudendal nerve, and the efferent limb via the inferior hemorrhoidal branch of the pudendal nerve. The reflex is integrated at the S2–4 cord level.[61,62,63,64] A normal response is a brisk contraction of the PFM akin to that of the quadriceps or biceps DTR. Hypo- and hyperreactivity are similarly defined.

A rectal evaluation is performed in a similar fashion (▶ Fig. 3.20). Palpation is to begin again at the ischial tuborosicty,

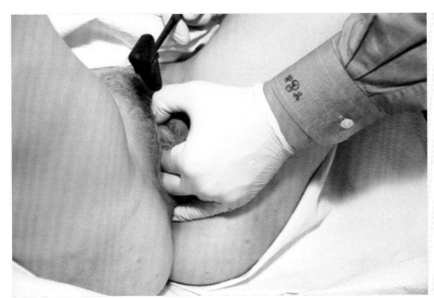

Fig. 3.19 Bulbospongiousus reflex.

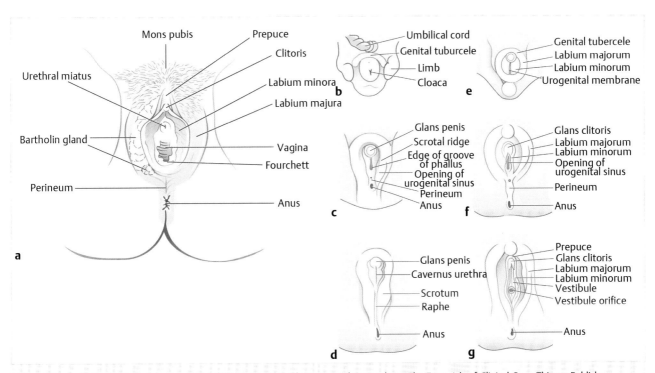

Fig. 3.20 a-g Anal palpation map. (From Reece EA, Barbieri RL, Obstetrics and Gynecology: The Essentials of Clinical Care, Thieme Publishers, Stuttgart: 2010. Used with permission.)

noting the origin of the superficial transverse perineal muscle for tissue continuity, crepitus, tenderness, and tone. The sacrotuberous ligament may be palpable as the clinician moves in a posterior medial fashion toward the anus, noting tissue continuity, crepitus, tenderness, and tone. The palpation continues in an anterior fashion toward the perineum, assessing the external anal sphincter for tissue continuity, crepitus, tenderness, and tone. And finally, the superficial transverse perineal muscle insertion and belly can be assessed for tissue continuity, crepitus, tenderness, and tone. The superficial anal reflex will then be assessed by gently stroking the external anal sphincter. An appropriate response is a slight reflexive contraction. The anal reflex assesses the integrity of the S3–5 spinal nerve root. The deep anal reflex is noted during initial rectal penetration, and a reflexive contraction of the PFM assessing the S5 nerve root conduction. MMT of the three layers is appropriate during a rectal examination, although discerning the three layers of musculature is more difficult due to the proximity of the anal canal to the origin of the musculature. Tinel testing can also be performed by gently running the palpating digit from the sacral sulci of S1–5, and in a similar fashion to that previously described, the pudendal nerve can be Tinel tested as well.

If there was a history of a fall, and landing on the coccyx, sacrococcygeal mobility testing would be appropriate. To do so, the patient is asked to assume the prone position, and having a pillow placed under the abdomen will assist in comfort. A well-lubricated digit is then gently inserted rectally to the metacarpal-phalangeal joint where it is then flexed so that the coccyx can be appreciated. The coccyx is then stabilized between this internal digit and the thumb, which is external. With firm, yet gentle pressure the coccyx is taken into a flexion and extension motion by the clinician flexing/extending the wrist. Sacrococcygeal rotations can be assessed by introducing a pronation-to-supination movement of the clinicians' forearm, and relative side-flexion is assessed with the clinician moving the forearm into radial and ulnar deviations. Appropriate motions should produce pain-free sacrococcygeal flexion and extension. Minor rotations and side-flexion movements may be present, and should be be pain free.

Clinical Note

During the course of the evaluation, consider where the patient is experiencing her pain; the proximal two-thirds of the vagina/rectum, or the distal one-third.

Were there other findings such as segmental hypomobility, positive prone knee flexion test or straight leg raising test, or a specific myotomal involvement that indicate a specific spinal segment(s)?

Using ▶ Table 3.1, were there correlational findings that share a common embryological origin?

If so, the provision of spinal mobilization with internal palpation can provide immediate confirmation of spinal involvement.

If during the course of the evaluation the clinician has reason to believe that the patient is suffering from a pain that involves a centrally sensitized spinal segment, the provision of a spinal mobilization with internal palpation may be appropriate. Such a finding may include deep vaginal pain, and perhaps a history of trauma and scarring. Remember, pain from the intraperitoneal pelvic viscera and proximal two-thirds of the vagina is transmitted via the uterovaginal and pelvic plexus, superior and inferior hypogastric plexus, and lumbar splanchnic nerves that arise from T11–12 to L4–5. To perform the spinal mobilization with internal palpation procedure, the clinician carefully isolates and palpates a region of the patient's pain. This region commonly involves a local muscle spasm, and patients are often quick to confirm that "You've found my pain." The mobilization is to be provided in a graded fashion (discussed in Chapter 5). If the clinician's suspicion was correct, both the patient and the clinician will note a palpable change in the tissue in question if a spasm is involved, and the patient will notice a reduction of pain. If the clinician is unable to perform a mobilization during internal palpation, the provision of a mobilization can occur in isolation, and then the painful tissue can be re-inspected. A change in the patient's pain, or tissue tone, is a strong indicator that there is a spinal dysfunction that is, at least in part, responsible for the patient's pain provocation and perpetuation. The side-lying mobilization shown in ▶ Fig. 3.21 and described in

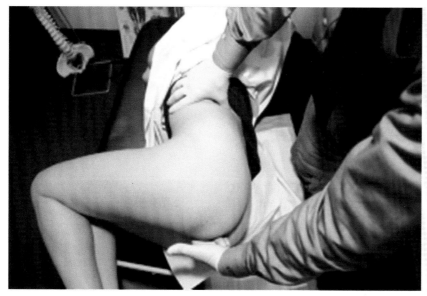

Fig. 3.21 Spinal mobilization with internal palpation.

Chapter 5 has been found to be very effective and efficient in providing pain relief. However, if the clinician does not possess the physical stature to perform an internal assessment while providing a spinal mobilization, the utilization of other spinal mobilizations such as a Central Posterior to Anterior (CPA) or a Unilateral Posterior to Anterior (UPA) will be equally useful. The purpose of maintaining the internal palpation while performing the spinal mobilization is to allow both the clinician and patient alike the opportunity to appreciate immediate resolution of the internal symptoms as a result of the spinal treatment.

References

[1] Khan KM, Cook JL, Maffulli N, Kannus P. Where is the pain coming from in tendinopathy? It may be biochemical, not only structural, in origin. Br J Sports Med 2000; 34: 81–83

[2] Khan KM, Cook JL, Taunton JE, Bonar F. Overuse tendinosis, not tendinitis part 1: a new paradigm for a difficult clinical problem. Phys Sportsmed 2000; 28: 38–48

[3] Ombregt L, Ed. (2003). A system of orthopaedic medicine (2nd ed.). Philadelphia, London: Churchill Livingstone

[4] Boyling JD, Ed. (2004). Grieve's modern manual therapy (3rd ed.). Edinburgh, London, New York, Oxford, Philadelphia, St. Louis, Sydney, Toronto: Churchill Livingstone

[5] Lukban JC, Parkin JV, Holzberg AS, Caraballo R, Kellogg-Spadt S, Whitmore KE. Interstitial cystitis and pelvic floor dysfunction: a comprehensive review. Pain Med 2001; 2: 60–71

[6] Carter JE. Diagnosis and treatment of the causes of chronic pelvic pain. J Am Assoc Gynecol Laparosc 1996; 3 Supplement: S5–S6

[7] Carter JE. A systematic history for the patient with chronic pelvic pain. JSLS 1999; 3: 245–252

[8] Tu FF, As-Sanie S, Steege JF. Musculoskeletal causes of chronic pelvic pain: a systematic review of diagnosis: part I. Obstet Gynecol Surv 2005a; 60: 379–385

[9] Tu FF, As-Sanie S, Steege JF. Musculoskeletal causes of chronic pelvic pain: a systematic review of existing therapies: part II. Obstet Gynecol Surv 2005b; 60: 474–483

[10] Tu FF, Fitzgerald CM, Kuiken T, Farrell T, Harden RN. Comparative measurement of pelvic floor pain sensitivity in chronic pelvic pain. Obstet Gynecol 2007; 110: 1244–1248

[11] Tu FF, Fitzgerald CM, Kuiken T, Farrell T, Norman Harden R. Vaginal pressure-pain thresholds: initial validation and reliability assessment in healthy women. Clin J Pain 2008; 24: 45–50

[12] Tu FF, Holt J, Gonzales J, Fitzgerald CM. Physical therapy evaluation of patients with chronic pelvic pain: a controlled study. Am J Obstet Gynecol 2008; 198: e1–e7

[13] Tu FF, Hahn D, Steege JF. Pelvic congestion syndrome-associated pelvic pain: a systematic review of diagnosis and management. Obstet Gynecol Surv 2010; 65: 332–340

[14] Lee SJ, Park JW. Follow-up evaluation of the effect of vaginal delivery on the pelvic floor. Dis Colon Rectum 2000; 43: 1550–1555

[15] Stuge B, Laerum E, Kirkesola G, Vøllestad N. The efficacy of a treatment program focusing on specific stabilizing exercises for pelvic girdle pain after pregnancy: a randomized controlled trial. Spine 2004; 29: 351–359

[16] Stuge B, Mørkved S, Dahl HH, Vøllestad N. Abdominal and pelvic floor muscle function in women with and without long lasting pelvic girdle pain. Man Ther 2006; 11: 287–296

[17] Stuge B. [Diagnosis and treatment of pelvic girdle pain] Tidsskr Nor Laegeforen 2010; 130: 2141–2145

[18] Gilroy AM, MacPherson BR, Ross LM, Eds. (2008). Atlas of anatomy. New York: Thieme

[19] Haines DE, Ed. (2008a). Neuroanatomy: An atlas of structures, sections and systems. Philadelphia: Lippincott Williams & Wilkins

[20] Jenkins DB, Ed. (2009). Hollinshead's functional anatomy of the limbs and back. Canada: Saunders

[21] Howard FM, Ed. (2000). Pelvic pain: Diagnosis & management. Philadelphia, Baltimore, New York, London, Buenos Aires, Hong Kong, Sydney & Tokyo: Lippincott Williams & Wilkins

[22] Cyriax J, Ed. (1982). Textbook of orthopaedic medicine. London, Philadelphia, Toronto, Sydney & Tokyo: WB Saunders & Bailliere Tindall

[23] Jantos M. Vulvodynia: a psychophysiological profile based on electromyographic assessment. Appl Psychophysiol Biofeedback 2008; 33: 29–38

[24] Laurent SM, Simons AD. Sexual dysfunction in depression and anxiety: conceptualizing sexual dysfunction as part of an internalizing dimension. Clin Psychol Rev 2009; 29: 573–585

[25] Greenman PE, Ed. (1996). Principles of manual medicine (4th ed.) Lippincott Williams & Wilkins

[26] Al-Eisa E, Egan D, Deluzio K, Wassersug R. Effects of pelvic asymmetry and low back pain on trunk kinematics during sitting: a comparison with standing. Spine 2006a; 31: E135–E143

[27] Al-Eisa E, Egan D, Deluzio K, Wassersug R. Effects of pelvic skeletal asymmetry on trunk movement: three-dimensional analysis in healthy individuals versus patients with mechanical low back pain. Spine 2006b; 31: E71–E79

[28] Al-Chaer ED, Lawand NB, Westlund KN, Willis WD. Pelvic visceral input into the nucleus gracilis is largely mediated by the postsynaptic dorsal column pathway. J Neurophysiol 1996; 76: 2675–2690

[29] Al-Chaer ED, Traub RJ. Biological basis of visceral pain: recent developments. Pain 2002b; 96: 221–225

[30] Giamberardino MA. Recent and forgotten aspects of visceral pain. Eur J Pain 1999a; 3: 77–92

[31] Meeus M, Nijs J. Central sensitization: a biopsychosocial explanation for chronic widespread pain in patients with fibromyalgia and chronic fatigue syndrome. Clin Rheumatol 2007; 26: 465–473

[32] Tu FF, As-Sanie S, Steege JF. Prevalence of pelvic musculoskeletal disorders in a female chronic pelvic pain clinic. J Reprod Med 2006; 51: 185–189

[33] Lawton S, Littlewood S. (2006). Vulval skin disease: Clinical features, assessment and management. Nursing Standard (Royal College of Nursing (Great Britain): 1987), 20(42), 57–63; quiz 64

[34] Lawton S. Anatomy and function of the skin, part 1. Nurs Times 2006a; 102: 26–27

[35] Lawton S. Anatomy and function of the skin. Part 2—the epidermis. Nurs Times 2006b; 102: 28–29

[36] Lawton S. Anatomy and function of the skin. Part 3—dermis and adjacent structures. Nurs Times 2006c; 102: 26–27

[37] Maitland G, Ed. (2005). Maitland's vertebral manipulation. Edinburgh, London, New York, Oxford, Philadelphia, St. Louis, Sydney, Toronto: Elisevier

[38] Damen L, Buyruk HM, Güler-Uysal F, Lotgering FK, Snijders CJ, Stam HJ. The prognostic value of asymmetric laxity of the sacroiliac joints in pregnancy-related pelvic pain. Spine 2002; 27: 2820–2824

[39] Lukban J, Whitmore K, Kellogg-Spadt S, Bologna R, Lesher A, Fletcher E. The effect of manual physical therapy in patients diagnosed with interstitial cystitis, high-tone pelvic floor dysfunction, and sacroiliac dysfunction. Urology 2001; 57 Suppl 1: 121–122

[40] Koury MJ, Scarpelli E. A manual therapy approach to evaluation and treatment of a patient with a chronic lumber nerve root irritation. Phys Ther 1994; 74: 548–560

[41] Herrera I, Ed. (2009). Ending female pain: A woman's manual. New York: Duplex Publishing

[42] Labat JJ, Riant T, Robert R et al. Diagnostic criteria for pudendal neuralgia by pudendal nerve entrapment (Nantes criteria). Neurourol Urodyn 2008; 27: 306–310

[43] Dietz HP. Levator trauma in labor: a challenge for obstetricians, surgeons and sonologists. Ultrasound Obstet Gynecol 2007; 29: 368–371

[44] Dietz HP, Gillespie AV, Phadke P. Avulsion of the pubovisceral muscle associated with large vaginal tear after normal vaginal delivery at term. Aust N Z J Obstet Gynaecol 2007; 47: 341–344

[45] Dietz HP, Shek C. Levator avulsion and grading of pelvic floor muscle strength. Int Urogynecol J Pelvic Floor Dysfunct 2008; 19: 633–636

[46] Dietz HP, Abbu A, Shek KL. The levator-urethra gap measurement: a more objective means of determining levator avulsion? Ultrasound Obstet Gynecol 2008; 32: 941–945

[47] Dietz HP, Kirby A. Modelling the likelihood of levator avulsion in a urogynaecological population. Aust N Z J Obstet Gynaecol 2010; 50: 268–272

[48] Dietz HP, Chantarasorn V, Shek KL. Levator avulsion is a risk factor for cystocele recurrence. Ultrasound Obstet Gynecol 2010; 36: 76–80

[49] Dietz HP, Bhalla R, Chantarasorn V, Shek KL. Avulsion of the puborectalis muscle is associated with asymmetry of the levator hiatus. Ultrasound Obstet Gynecol 2011; 37: 723–726

[50] Mercer S. Anatomy in practice: The ischiorectal fossae. NZ J of Physiotherapy 2005; 33: 61–64

[51] Padilla LA, Radosevich DM, Milad MP. Limitations of the pelvic examination for evaluation of the female pelvic organs. Int J Gynaecol Obstet 2005; 88: 84–88

[52] Kearney R, Miller JM, Delancey JO. Interrater reliability and physical examination of the pubovisceral portion of the levator ani muscle, validity comparisons using MR imaging. Neurourol Urodyn 2006; 25: 50–54

[53] Kearney R, Miller JM, Ashton-Miller JA, DeLancey JO. Obstetric factors associated with levator ani muscle injury after vaginal birth. Obstet Gynecol 2006; 107: 144–149

[54] Ventegodt S, Thegler S, Andreasen T et al. Clinical holistic medicine: psychodynamic short-time therapy complemented with bodywork. A clinical follow-up study of 109 patients. ScientificWorldJournal 2006; 6: 2220–2238

[55] Hurd WW, Wyckoff ET, Reynolds DB, Amesse LS, Gruber JS, Horowitz GM. Patient rotation and resolution of unilateral cornual obstruction during hysterosalpingography. Obstet Gynecol 2003; 101: 1275–1278

[56] Carriere B, Markel FC, Eds. (2006). The pelvic floor. New York: Thieme

[57] Maffulli N, Ewen SW, Waterston SW, Reaper J, Barrass V. Tenocytes from ruptured and tendinopathic achilles tendons produce greater quantities of type III collagen than tenocytes from normal achilles tendons. An in vitro model of human tendon healing. Am J Sports Med 2000; 28: 499–505

[58] Maffulli N, Wong J. Rupture of the Achilles and patellar tendons. Clin Sports Med 2003; 22: 761–776

[59] Maffulli N, Kenward MG, Testa V, Capasso G, Regine R, King JB. Clinical diagnosis of Achilles tendinopathy with tendinosis. Clin J Sport Med 2003; 13: 11–15

[60] Maffulli N, Wong J, Almekinders LC. Types and epidemiology of tendinopathy. Clin Sports Med 2003; 22: 675–692

[61] Amarenco G, Bayle B, Ismael SS, Kerdraon J. Bulbocavernosus muscle responses after suprapubic stimulation: analysis and measurement of suprapubic bulbocavernosus reflex latency. Neurourol Urodyn 2002; 21: 210–213

[62] Larson W, Ed. (2002). Anatomy: Development, function, clinical correlations. Philadelphia, London, New York, St. Louis, Sydney & Toronto: Saunders

[63] Nout YS, Leedy GM, Beattie MS, Bresnahan JC. Alterations in eliminative and sexual reflexes after spinal cord injury: defecatory function and development of spasticity in pelvic floor musculature. Prog Brain Res 2006; 152: 359–372

[64] Shafik A, Shafik I, El-Sibai O. Effect of vaginal distension on anorectal function: identification of the vagino-anorectal reflex. Acta Obstet Gynecol Scand 2005; 84: 225–229

4 Interpretation

Serious pathology does occur. It is appropriate for the patients suffering from a pelvic pain to have undergone an evaluation by their medical doctor to rule out the presence of disease, ailment, and structural injury. Once overall health has been confirmed, the following interpretation is helpful in assisting the patient who is suffering.

Learning Objectives

- The clinician will recognize the subtle indicators that allow the formation of a functional diagnosis of the patient with pelvic pain.
- The clinician will construct a treatment protocol based upon his or her findings during the evaluation.
- The clinician will paraphrase his or her findings regarding the patient and relay them to the management team.

Unlike the evaluation of the axial spine or peripheral joints, the clinician evaluating the patient with pelvic pain must often make functional assessments based on the series of findings that indicate where and why the patient is suffering. The findings may be parallel in nature indicating a relationship. An example of this would be the patient presenting with the following history:

- Initial diagnosis of irritable bowel disease
- Secondary diagnosis of "interstitial cystitis"
- Third diagnosis of pudendal neuralgia
- History:
  - Six months ago the patient had a forceful bowel movement, after becoming dehydrated after a night of alcohol consumption.
  - This lead to persistent malaise throughout the gastrointestinal tract.
  - She states that she was told that her pelvic pain is due to damage of the pudendal nerve and it is a life-long condition and that she should "get used to it."
  - She continues by stating that she feels abandoned by the medical community and spends wakeful nights "researching" pelvic pain on her smartphone.
  - The more she "learns" the more fearful she becomes. She senses that her symptoms are worsening monthly.
- Current symptoms:
  - Abdominal malaise
  - Pain with bowel movements
  - Dyspareunia
  - Discomfort, with palpable spasms throughout the abdominal musculature below the umbilicus
  - Burning sensation throughout "urethra" and "bladder"
  - Sensation of sitting on a golf ball
- Current presentation:
  - Patient sits in hyperkyphotic fashion
  - Angle of declination is 45 degrees
  - Apical respiration pattern
  - Constant, low-grade writhing in waiting room and evaluation room

- Active range of motion (AROM) of spine is grossly limited from T10 to L3 with side flexion; flexion is appropriate and extension is limited to 10%
- Tests:
  - Positive prone knee flexion with palpable fasciculation
  - Positive hypomobility of central posterior-to-anterior (CPA) at T10 to L3
  - Increased tone of bilateral iliopsoas
  - Palpable muscle "tender points" throughout abdominal musculature below umbilicus
  - Provision of CPA at T11 to L2, grade II
    - 90% reduction of patient's symptoms at abdomen and saddle region
    - Elimination of muscle "tender points" throughout the abdominal musculature
    - 75% reduction of iliopsoas tone
- Commonalities:
  - Positive prone knee flexion (L1–3)
  - Iliopsoas tenderness
  - Bladder, colon, vagina, uterus, ureter, and ovaries have same embryologic derivation
- Diagnosis:
  - Central sensitization of T11 to L2, with convergence and symptom propagation to segmentally common viscus and secondary muscle tender points
- Explanation:
  - The distal colon and vagina have a common embryological derivation.
  - The segmental distribution of muscle spasm/malaise from T12 to L2 is the lower abdominal region.
  - Anxiety regarding the rapid onset of a pelvic pain, loss of comfortable intimacy, and perseveration over a "life-long injury," coupled with gross fatigue due to poor sleep, led to a hyperkyphotic posture.
  - Patient's history did not indicate an internal pelvic examination as appropriate at this time.
- Treatment:
  - Postural education
  - Postural re-conditioning exercises
  - Education of the patient regarding the interaction of the nervous system, referred pain, and resultant tenderness, and of the interaction her actions and postures will have in perpetuating or eliminating her pain.

As noted above, there were no glaring findings that led the clinician to the diagnosis. What occurred was the summarization of commonalities during the course of the evaluation, followed by the application of a segmental mobilization at a grade II to these segments in an attempt to address the patient's pain. Following the application of the mobilizations, the findings of abdominal tender points, increased iliopsoas tone, and subjective symptoms were reassessed. Any reduction of symptoms strongly indicates the involvement of that/those spinal segment(s), and a phenomenon of central sensitization.

What were the patient's primary complaints during the history taking component of the evaluation? Did they indicate a region of the body that was involved? Urological? Bowel?

Gynecologic? Or did the symptoms represent allodynia or hyperalgesia? If so, was the pain local or regional and are the symptoms progressing from one system to another? If the symptoms appear to be "progressing" from one system to another, are those structures related embryologically?

If the symptoms were isolated to a single aspect of the urological, bowel, or gynecologic system, was there any aspect of the history or the clinical testing that indicated a reason for this pain? Were there any segmental losses of motion during the active lumbar screening that reflect the viscus' embryological derivation? If so, did a manipulation/mobilization locally positively influence these symptoms? If so, then the patient is likely suffering from a facilitated segment and is an appropriate patient for physical therapy care. If not, then further testing may be indicated, a referral to a gynecologist, urologist, or colorectal specialist, or the patient may possibly be insincere.

Did the history and clinical findings indicate a local nerve entrapment? If so, were these symptoms alterable with manipulations/mobilizations to the spine, or local transverse friction massage to the pelvic musculotendinous structures?

Were there any scars that impede motion, entrap peripheral nerves, perpetuate pain, limit or prevent complete closure during internal manual muscle testing (MMT)? If addressing the scar(s), were the patient's symptoms eliminated? If so, then the clinician can deduce that the scarring was a considerable factor in pain initiation and propagation. Addressing the appropriate spinal segment may further alleviate the patient's pain, as the segment will likely have become sensitized due to the persistent noxious stimulation from the scar.

Were any of the special tests positive? If so, do they implicate a region that requires additional testing? Or does local treatment to the region alleviate the patient's symptoms?

Discerning findings of the evaluation:

- Were there active motions of the spine that reproduce symptoms that indicate a closer evaluation of that region of the spine?

- Was there local, segmental hypomobility of the spine that reflects the patient's symptoms, a somatic representation of embryogenesis?
- Segmental weaknesses suggest a closer inspection of the suspected spinal level. Is there a correlation of segmental weakness to neuroanatomy with presenting symptoms?
- Neural tension testing is reflective of the overall mobility of the nervous system. Are there any restrictions that relate to the level of spinal integration?
  ○ Are there any fasciculations with prone knee flexion (PKF)?
- Does the hip have any restrictions? Does passive movement reproduce the patient's pain?
- CPAs and unilateral posterior-to-anterior (UPA)s: do they move appropriately? Do they reproduce pain along the suspected segment? Do they eliminate pain, spasm, or neurological symptoms?
- During the course of the pelvic evaluation, was there any pain while assessing the "pelvic map"?
- Were there any asymmetries in strength right versus left, and between the layers one, two, and three?
- Was there any scarring within the birth canal?
- Was there a lack of muscle bulk, indicating breach of musculature along any of the pelvic floor muscles?
- Was there a positive Tinel test of any of the sacral nerves, or the pudendal nerves?
- Was the bulbospongiosus symmetrical, latent or hyper-reflexive?
  ○ Does this correlate with any of the SIJ findings?
- Was there the presence of the distal rectum, bladder, or uterus within the vaginal canal?
  ○ Did the mobilization of this structure improve contraction grade of the PFM?
- Was the anterior SIJ ligament painful and/or noted to have crepitus along its length?

5 Management

It is globally acknowledged that the treatment strategies for patients suffering with pelvic pain conditions are to be multi-faceted. It is through the integration of neurological, movement, segmental, physiological, and scar assessment, and the assessment/modification of the patient's behavior, perception of pain, locus of control, sleeping habits, eating habits, and perseveration on pain that a clinician can be successful at eliminating the patient's pain.

> **Learning Objectives**
>
> - The clinician will demonstrate tissue-specific treatment to the patient with pelvic pain.
> - The clinician will defend his or her choice of treatment.
> - The clinician will support his or her decision to treat externally or internally the patient suffering with a pelvic pain.
>   - The clinician will appraise the patient's progression regarding pain amelioration based upon the treatment the patient has received.

It has been the observation of many authors that the aggressive, direct treatment of vulvar vestibulitis and other pelvic pain conditions may in fact heighten the pain experience and response through neural hyperplasia, and serve as a perpetuating factor increasing these painful conditions.[1] It is with this in mind that the clinician will best serve the patient by not promoting or encouraging pain during the course of the evaluation and subsequent treatments, and in its place offer the patient a means of healing that is pain free and directly addresses the cause(s) of the pain and muscle spasms.[2]

The purpose of a treatment is to accurately address the tissue at fault in a fashion that will impart a direct and beneficial impact on that tissue.[3,4] This necessitates a thorough and specific evaluation be completed and interpreted correctly utilizing a sound understanding of the various interactions of the nervous system and the relative joints and musculature in the formation of a functional diagnosis to maximize the patient's healing experience. All treatments are to be as gentle as possible, but as strong as necessary.[3,4]

Painful conditions of the pelvis can be managed in many ways, depending on the source of the pain. A list of elements of the etiology of pain in each case will help in choosing the appropriate management method, and may be composed by answering the following questions:
- What structures appear to be involved?
- Was there a segmental restriction?
  - What is the embryological level of derivation of the structure represented by the patient's symptoms?
- Are there scars and are they mobile?
  - Do they reproduce the patient's pain?
- What dermatome innervates the region the patient indicates as painful?
- What peripheral nerves innervate the specified region and does the history offer a rationale as to why a peripheral nerve may have become entrapped?
- What somatic structures refer pain that represent the patient's pain pattern?
- What is the nature of the symptoms?
  - Do spasms dominate the condition, or hyperalgesia/allodynia?
- History of pelvic trauma

5.1 Biopsychosocial Treatment: Education

At the end of the evaluation, the clinician should have a series of findings, where a pattern of segmental involvement can be determined. If so, then treatment involving a posterior-to-anterior mobilization can be introduced at that level in an attempt to assess theoretical accuracy. If the symptoms are altered, the clinician will have a strong indication of neurological involvement.

> **Hierarchy of Treatment**
>
> - Biopsychosocial factors
>   - Somatization
>   - Perseveration
>   - Anxiety
> - Neurological
>   - Referred pain
>   - Centralization, convergence, and sensitization
> - Joint festrictions
>   - Facet inflammation/referred pain
>   - Internal derangement of hip
>   - Arthropathy
> - Scar presence and restrictions
>   - Abdominal
>   - Perineal
>   - Hip
> - Muscle imbalance and generalized weakness
>   - Postural faults
>   - Sitting
>   - Standing
> - Muscle spasms, facial restrictions, and trigger points

Utilizing the hierarchy noted here, all treatments are to begin with education aimed initially at attaining and maintaining appropriate neutral spinal alignment as outlined by McKenzie.[5] This will serve many purposes: (1) it will minimize the strain throughout the dural structures, (2) it will serve as a means for the clinician to assess the patient's willingness to participate in her own health care, and (3), it will empower the patient to self-correct, and decrease the hyperkyphotic alignment that reflects a state of hypervigilance while decreasing the secondary muscle tenderness associated with this posture. This format has been shown to be effective at facilitating the healing process for all pelvic pain patients, regardless of central involvement. The assumption is that change of locus of control from passive recipient of pain to active participant in healing will lead to a more positive outcome.[3,4,6,7]

Up to 85% of patients suffering with a chronic pelvic pain will have musculoskeletal dysfunction and postural changes including scoliosis and pelvic rotation. Abnormal postures have been found to increase muscular tension and spasms with subsequent muscle shortening that further aggravates the patient's pain, resulting in persistent, perpetuated pain cycles.[8,9]

A significant portion of the treatment regimen for the pelvic pain patient may be to optimize patient's postures during common activities of daily living. Doing so will assist in her overall healing process.[10,11,12,13,14,15,16,17] Postural training is imperative for efficiently healing the individual with spine-facilitated pain. Stresses and strains associated with postures, especially flexion, will increase the production of glial and plial scar formation and concomitant fluid-filled cavities.[10,11,12,13,14,15] Due to the arrangement of the spinal anatomy, deformation of the spinal canal will lead to deformation of the internal structures of the canal. As an example, it was found that the S2 nerve root was tensioned, or strained 16% during a combination of cervical and lumbar flexion: the slouched position.[10,11,12,13,14,15] The correction of a patient's posture will have a twofold benefit: (1) it will minimize the aforementioned neuromechanical strains and (2) it will afford the patient the opportunity to be an active participant in their healing process, thereby empowering themselves to heal.

Intervertebral disk pressures are directly related to the alignment of the spine to the thigh and the angle of the hip and knees.[3,4,10,11,12,13,14,15,16] Less than optimal spinal alignment will increase focal stresses, restrict spinal capsular capacious qualities, and impede imbibition (the means to which the spinal structures receive nourishment). Imbibition dictates the need for movement, and this was noted by Harrison and colleagues by the overwhelming preference for "adjustable" chairs to meet this need.[10,13,14,15,16] Harrison and co-workers further reported the reduction of lower back pain, and the reduction of paraspinal muscle activity and forward inclination of the head, when a lumbar support was utilized in conjunction with firm foam as the material on which one sits, along with the use of armrests.[11,16,18] A correction of prolonged, static positions will further limit the detrimental compressive forces to which the intervertebral disks are subject. This will reduce the likelihood a primary disk lesion, and if the patient's symptoms are either directly or indirectly related to neural irritation, then the simple practice of attaining and maintaining appropriate, erect postures will assist in the long-term healing process.

Postural dysfunctions, as they relate to the pelvic pain patient, may be due to:
- Childhood injuries
- Structural malformation: scoliosis, short-leg syndrome, hemipelvis
- Poor ergonomics
- Recreations activities
- Frequent wearing of high heels
- Sedentary lifestyle
- Constant sitting in poorly designed chairs and sofas
- Pregnancy
- Breast feeding positions
- Trauma: motor vehicle accident, sport, etc.
- Poor breathing patterns
- Illness or disorders: emphysema, asthma, chronic fatigue syndrome
- Surgical adhesions
- Pelvic laxity

As the patient is progressing through the rehabilitation program, it is appropriate that the clinician be immediately present to offer gentle words of encouragement, and postural corrections as necessary. Often the patient will require verbal assurance that the malaise of exercise is appropriate and necessary, and is to be considered as distinct from the pain she has been suffering. All too often, the patient suffering will associate any local pain as a regression of their status regardless of origin, exercise induced or otherwise. Determining the factors that motivate the individual will assist in their desire to participate in the re-conditioning program. Discuss with the patient what their goals are, and attempt to introduce movements, exercises, and activities that meet those goals.

5.2 Biopsychosocial Treatment: Cognitive Behavioral Therapy

Clinicians must be aware that depression and anxiety commonly accompany patients who suffer from pelvic pain. It is often quite difficult to determine what the cause is, and what the effect is. It is further known that patients with pelvic pain will demonstrate "health care seeking behavior"; however, a direct link to psychological and physical disease has yet to be found.[19] Williams et al compared women with chronic pelvic pain with healthy women, analyzing their depression, anxiety, and sexual dysfunction using the following scales: Beck Depression Inventory (BDI), Beck Anxiety Inventory (BAI), Spielberger Trait Anxiety Inventory (STAI), and the Golombok Rust Inventory of Sexual Satisfaction (GRISS).[19] The findings concluded that those with chronic pelvic pain had significantly higher BDI and BAI scores when compared with the normal population, and the GRISS score was also found to be significantly higher in those with chronic pelvic pain. Those suffering from chronic pelvic pain also were found to have greater difficulty communicating with loved ones. They often demonstrate avoidance behaviors and they state that they have a decreased sense of sensuality and sexuality. There was no difference found in reported relative to anorgasmia,[20] indicating appropriate physiological function and absence of dysfunction.

Behavioral modification is imperative in the treatment of those with chronic pelvic pain. The neurological systems, both central and peripheral, must be desensitized through a progressive introduction of movement activities that do not provoke pain. This, in part, can be accomplished by reducing joint restrictions with joint-specific mobilizations and allowing the patients to partake in movement and activity. Somatization is the propensity to experience and report somatic symptoms that have no pathophysiological explanation, and to misattribute them to disease and then seek medical attention.[21,22] Patients with a catastrophic perspective have a greater rated disability index, greater rated disability, and greater health care utilization as compared with those who are unaffected. Anxiety toward activity, intimate or otherwise, produces a state of hypervigilance, which in turn facilitates greater muscle tension and pain, and perpetuates the cycle of activity avoidance and pain behaviors.[23] "Nonanatomic" pelvic pain syndromes do not

Table 5.1 Pain management techniques

Goal	Intervention
Control pain	Relaxation techniques
	Stress management
	"Self-talk"
	Pain coping strategies
	Pain attributions
	Distraction techniques
Reduce disability	Progressive activities
	Pain behavior modification
	Re-employment
	Treat substance abuse
Promote wellness/improve lifestyle	Eating behaviors/nutrition
	Physical exercise
	Sleeping
Treat psychological morbidity	Treat depression and anxiety
	Abuse survivors
	Couples/family counseling
	Sex therapy

respond well to biomedicine, but they do respond better with psychosomatic treatments.[24]

Continual passive movement and movement in general have been shown to facilitate healing of synovial joints, and the regeneration of hyaline cartilage, in addition to the maintenance of appropriate joint characteristics necessary for normal function. This is explained by: (1) improved fluid dynamics, (2) stimulation of mechanoreceptors to obtund pain, (3) prevention/lessoning of restrictive/painful adhesions, and (4), possibly, the promotion of the formation of a pseudodisk.[25]

Cognitive behavioral psychological pain management techniques, as outlined by Howard,[8] are detailed in ▶ Table 5.1.

5.3 Neurological and Joint Treatments: Manipulations and Mobilizations

Manipulation is an ancient art of healing dating back to the time of Hippocrates, and it has been used intermittently by the medical community in the treatment of pain, swelling, and spasms.[26] Ancient Chinese, Egyptian, and Greek medical accounts note the change in respiration rate, arterial pulse, and reduction of muscle tone with the application of mobilizations to the bony pelvis.[27,28] Manipulation and mobilizations have been found to be equally effective in the eradication of pain and restoration of function.[29,30] Research performed on sheep has demonstrated that short and fast thrusts have been found to produce larger adjacent segmental motion, and research that utilized longer pulse durations actually caused greater local motion at the segmental contact point.[31] Therefore, we will be discussing the use of manipulations and mobilizations throughout this textbook.

Utilizing spinal mobilizations or manipulations in the treatment of pelvic pain is not a unique concept. According to Jamison et al, 11% of the chiropractic profession of Australia has

utilized spinal adjustments to manage their patients with pelvic pain.[32] Browning found spinal manipulation to be an underused treatment modality in the treatment of pelvic pain.[33] According to Weiss, a common cause of persistent pain after neural decompression surgery revolves around the sensitized nerve, connective tissue, muscles, and ligaments that had initially predisposed the nerve to injury and then remained the dominant problem following surgery.[34] What is unique, however, is the application of spinal mobilizations as directed by embryological derivation, and the concurrent treatments that will assist in the overall management of the patient with pelvic pain. By mapping the patient's pain and symptomology, physical presentation, and positive clinical testing maneuvers, and then tracing back the viscus in question, the clinician will know where along the spine each treatment is to be applied. Take the following into consideration as a common presentation:

- Patient A reports pain deep within the rectum.
- Active motions of the spine demonstrate local hypomobility of T10 to L3.
- Segmental, arthrokinematic, testing confirms local hypomobility of T10 to L3.
- Prone knee flexion test is positive; fasciculations are noted.
- The clinician can cross-reference the patient's history, with the tests shown in ▶ Table 5.2, and determine that treatment via mobilizations can be initiated at T12 to L2.

Spinal mobilizations have been shown to be effective in the treatment of acute and subacute lower back pain. Biomechanically, mobilizations/manipulations facilitate the restoration of segmental mobility and the restoration of function[34,35] through the repeated loading of the spinal connective tissues. Decreased resistance to segmental, arthrokinematic movement is due to creep deformation and microfailure of tight connective tissue.[35,36] This has been achieved after 9 minutes of end-range posterior-anterior mobilizations in *a*symptomatic subjects. Single-treatment sessions involving two minutes of central posterior to anterior spinal mobilizations demonstrate minimal osteokinematic improvements of motion. It is only via continued treatments and the postural/lifestyle education that actual improvements in spinal osteokinematic motions can be appreciated.[35,36]

Beneficial physiological responses to spinal mobilizations and manipulations include the transient decrease of motorneuronal activity. As reported by Dishman, the facilitation of motor-evoked potentials in the gastronomies was noted after a spinal mobilization/manipulation; it was not noted in those who had assumed a nonmanipulative side-lying position.[37,38,39,40,41] It was further found that group Ia, Ib, II, and IV afferents responded in a graded fashion to the velocity, magnitude, and direction of a vertebral loading. Stimulation of group Ib, III, and IV muscle afferents actually exerted an inhibitory effect on alpha motor neurons. Thoracic and lumbar spinal mobilizations and manipulations have been shown to be safe and effective in treating a variety of pain conditions. The risks involved with performing a thoracolumbar manipulation have been studied and the rate of injury has been found to be 1 in 3.7 million.[42] Considering these findings, the mobilizations that will be discussed here are the CPA variety as outlined by Maitland, Cyriax et al.[3,43] Other mobilization techniques have shown to be effective as well; however, covering all the various techniques is beyond the scope of the textbook.

Table 5.2 Embryological origin of selected organs and joints

Organ/Joint	C3	C4	T6	T7	T8	T9	T10	T11	T12	L1	L2	L3	L4	L5	S1	S2	S3	S4	S5	Co1	Co2
SCJ	X	X																			
Pancreas				X	X																
Liver						X															
Gall Bladder			X	X	X	X	X														
Stomach/duodenum				X	X	X	X														
Small intestine						X	X														
Epididymis							X														
Colon: ascending							X	X	X	X											
Kidney							X	X	X	X											
Appendix							X	X	X	X											
Ureter								X	X	X											
Bladder fundus								X	X	X											
Uterine fundus								X	X	X											
Bladder Neck								X	X	X											
Vagina								X	X	X											
Suprarenal gland								X	X	X											
Ovary/testes								X	X	X											
Colon; flexure										X	X	X									
Colon; sigmoid																	X	X	X		
Prostate																X	X	X	X		
Urethra																X	X	X	X		
Rectum																	X	X	X		

In the provision of mobilizations/manipulations, the clinician need not be concerned with producing an audible "click." It has been shown that cavitation is not an essential component of a manipulation or mobilization.[44] As long as the contraindications are respected, the provision of a mobilization/manipulation is a viable treatment choice. Rationale for the provision of a mobilization/manipulation is the presence of a localized muscle spasm, or a restriction of movement at a joint and or the presence of pain.[45] Improvements of range of motion and reduction of muscle spasms after the provision of a mobilization/manipulation have been noted regardless of symptom duration, and those suffering will often experience the greatest improvements.[46,47,48] When performing a mobilization or manipulation, the clinician must take care to determine the effected side, as a compressive event, further joint loading, will occur on the contralateral side to that being treated.[49]

Joint dysfunction is often the result of adhesions and muscle contractures, and poor stabilization capacities of the ligaments and muscles. The application of a mobilization and manipulation improves local osteokinematic properties of a joint and is essential for rapid absorption of scar tissue, and affords better structural organization of the healing tissues.[50,51] Mobilization-induced hypoalgesia has been demonstrated in numerous studies on humans, indicating that mobilizing an area of injury and the area proximal to injury reduces hyperalgesia.[52,53,54,55,56,57] Stimulation of the central nervous system (CNS) will induce a release of endogenous chemicals from cells in pain control circuits via the stimulation of periventricular gray matter (PVG), periaqueductal gray (PAG), or the nucleus raphe magnus with the resultant release of enkephalin or monoamines producing analgesia.[58] Furthermore, mobilizations effectively lead to a bilateral activation of descending inhibitory pathways that result in a reduction of hyperalgesia, and sympathoexcitatory effects of the treatment were noted in changes of skin conductance and cutaneous blood flux.[59] The reduction of hyperalgesia by joint mobilization and manipulation involves the release of 5-hydroxytryptamine (5-HT) serotoninergic and alpha-2 noradrenergic receptors in the spinal cord. 5-HT receptors are for neurotransmitter and peripheral signal mediator serotonin. 5-HT receptors are located on the cell membrane of nerve cells and other cell types including smooth muscles in animals, and they mediate the effects of serotonin as the endogenous ligand. 5-HT receptors also affect the release of other neurotransmitters including glutamate, dopamine, and gamma-amino butyric acid (GABA). Data from research indicate that it is the activation of nonopioid pathways that are involved with descending inhibition through serotonin and noradrenaline that produce the analgesia.[37,38,39,40,41,54,55,56,60]

Joint mobilization and manipulation also activate muscle spindle and golgi tendon organ primary afferent fibers, which may inhibit the alpha-motor neuron and reduce muscle spasms and hyperalgesia. Pain is initiated in the Type IV receptor system, and it is carried to the brain via the anterolateral spinal tracts. These tracts can be modulated by all peripheral and/or articular mechanoreceptors. Activation of the peripheral mechanoreceptors by joint or soft-tissue manipulation will reduce the presynaptic inhibition of nociceptive afferent activity and lead to pain suppression. The alleviation of muscle spasms is likely due to the stimulation of Type I and II mechanoreceptors within the spinal joints themselves. The result is the modulation of activity involving the fusimotor muscle spindle loop system.[26]

There is growing evidence as to the efficacy of spinal mobilization and manipulation therapy in the treatment of pain regarding long-term potentiation (LTP) and long-term depression (LTD). Spinal mobilization/manipulative therapy are thought to address the LTP, which is known to be reversible, within a sensitized pain-signaling segment of the spine.[61] LTD has been noted to occur in the dorsal horn neurons after low-frequency stimulation of A-delta afferent fibers and has further been shown to reverse the LTP established by C-fiber activation of those same dorsal horn neurons. The LTD has been observed to last for days, and the improved biomechanics through spinal mobilization/manipulative therapy may allow for the restoration of normal activities, which will facilitate central de-sensitization.[62] The phenomenon of neuroplasticity[63] has been noted to occur as a response to a variety of internal and external demands made on the nervous system inclusive of mobilizations/manipulations. Spinal mobilization/manipulation therapy appears to be effective through the stimulation of A-beta, A-delta, and C-fibers and less for the mechanical "breaking of adhesions." It is under this premise that the utilization of a mobilization or manipulation of the spine is found be effective in treating those patients who are suffering from pain due to a facilitated segment, central sensitization. Effects of mobilization/manipulation on local dorsal horn-mediated inhibition of A-delta and C-fibers have been noted as a potential hypoalgesic mechanism and have been found to have both local and peripheral effects in the lumbar spine; A-delta has also been found to be mediated with stationary bicycle riding and lumbar extension exercises.[52] This has been noted as a result of local antiinflammatory[57] and decreased electromyography (EMG) activity.[46,47,48,64]

> ### Clinical Note
>
> LTP is due to plastic deformation of the dorsal horn.
>   LTD is what occurs as a result of reversing the plastic deformation.

Mobilization and manipulative spinal therapy offers segmental hypoalgesia and has been found to be more effective at alleviating pain mediated by C-fibers than exercise alone.[52] Grade III mobilizations have been noted to increase sympathetic efferent activity of a normal, pain-free upper limb when performed at C5 as compared with lesser gradations of mobilizations,[65] resulting in a greater response of sympathetic efferent activity.[66] The result of spinal mobilizations was the production of a hypoalgesic effect as revealed by increased pressure pain thresholds on the side of treatment ($p = 0.0001$) and decreased resting visual analogue scale scores ($p = 0.049$). The treatment technique also produced a sympathoexcitatory effect with an increase in skin conductance ($p < 0.002$) and a decrease in skin temperature ($p \leq 0.02$). There was a decrease in superficial neck flexor muscle activity ($p < 0.0002$) at the lower levels of a staged craniocervical flexion test. This could imply facilitation of the deep neck flexor muscles with a decreased need for co-activation of the superficial neck flexors. The combination of all

findings would support the proposal that mobilization/manipulation may, at least initially, exert part of its influence via activation of the PAG.[67]

In the medical profession of pain management, the superior hypogastric blockade has been found to be useful in the treatment of pelvic pain that originates from the uterus and upper vagina, bladder, prostate, urethra, seminal vesicles, testes, and ovaries; or pain due to radiation, pain that is sympathetically maintained (after rectal anastomoses, abdomino-perineal resection), or pain that is from chronic pelvic inflammatory conditions. An inferior hypogastric plexus injection has been useful for the treatment of perianal pain of malignant or sympathetically mediated origin, burning, and urgency.[68,69,70]

Considering the beneficial effects of imparting a mobilization and manipulation on target tissues, the trained clinician will have a treatment option for patients that will address the aforementioned pain characteristics above and beyond that of an injection.[26,52,54,55,56,67] In the treatment of a painful muscle spasm of the pelvic floor musculature (PFM), the clinician will want to consider the involved anatomy. Is there a common spinal segment(s) that the patient's pain pattern suggests, and that the clinician was able to confirm through the evaluation and testing process? If so, provide the mobilization to the suspected segments, and reassess the patient's status. The clinician should also recall that sympathetic outflow to the pelvic viscera originates in the hypogastric plexus. If the evaluation was negative, the clinician may choose to initiate treatment at the segments that involve the hypogastric plexus. If the segments that compose the hypogastric plexus are the source of the spasms and pain, upon completion of the mobilization, both the patient and the clinician will note the immediate alleviation of her painful spasms without having to compromise her modesty or utilize painful massage or dilation techniques.

Menstrual pain associated with primary dysmenorrhea may be alleviated with treatment of motion segment restrictions of the lumbosacral spine with a drop-table technique.[71] The theory behind treatment of the lumbosacral spine in treating dysmenorrhea is based upon the neurological connection between uterine function and the sacral nerve roots. Aberrant joint motions can be corrected resulting in sympathetic response inhibiting uterine contraction and increased blood flow to the pelvic region. An alternate theory suggests that spinal manipulation of the lumbosacral spine will interfere with referred pain originating from the same pelvic nerve pathways associated with uterine dysfunction and primary dysmenorrhea.[71] Spinal manipulation affects the sacral position, which will decrease tension on the broad ligament of the uterus and pelvic nerve roots, possibly alleviating menstrual pain.[72,73,74] Holtzman et al considered spinal manipulation to be effective in the treatment of dysmennorhea.[71]

In a study by the Maigne et al in which massage and manipulation were used in the treatment of coccydynia and compared with a group that received external shortwave (magnetic field) physical therapy, more improvement was noted via a visual analogue scale (VAS) and pain questionnaire in the massage and manipulation group at one month. The 6-month findings, however, demonstrated modest improvements at best.[75] The lack of carryover from the first to the sixth month illustrates the need for greater attention to be given to the patient with regard to other propagating factors, including: perseveration on pain,

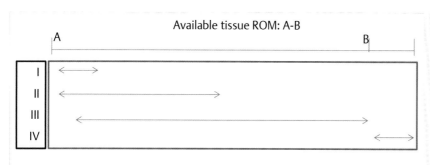

Available tissue ROM: A-B

Fig. 5.1 Mobilization grade and available tissue range of motion.

postural proclivities, poor sleeping or dietary habits, and/or poor to nonexistent activity in addition to the cause of the muscle spasm and pain. It is through the integration of various treatment strategies that the physical therapy profession ensures that its patients will obtain the most benefit.[76]

To assist in determining where to further evaluate and treat a patient with pelvic pain, consider which aspect of the urogenital system is involved. The sensory information from the external genitals is carried by the sacral afferent parasympathetic system, whereas those of the internal genitals is carried by the hypogastric, pelvic, and vagus nerves that transmit information regarding the uterus and vagina.[68,69,70,77] Therefore, treatment whose purpose is the alleviation of pain at the external genitalia is to be directed at the sacrum and sacral nerves, whereas that which involves the internal genitalia is to be directed at the segments involving the hypogastric, pelvic, and vagus nerves. Therefore, the clinician must take note of the location of the patient's pain during the history and pelvic examination. Symptoms that are reproduced along the distal third of the vagina or anus may benefit from a mobilization or manipulation to the sacral spine and sacroiliac joints (SIJs), whereas symptoms that are reproduced in the deeper two-thirds of the vagina and anus during the pelvic examination may best be treated with thoracolumbar mobilizations and manipulations.

5.4 Mobilization Technique

The application of a mobilization is to begin with a segmental stretch assessment, centrally and unilaterally, one segment at a time. This testing procedure, like the active and passive motion testing during the evaluation, will assess: the patient's ability to tolerate a local, segmental movement, pain/symptom provocation, pain/symptom resolution, and joint stability. In determining whether or not to apply a central mobilization or a unilateral mobilization, the clinician will perform a stretch articulation and segmental movement assessment. If, during the evaluation, the clinician finds a particular segment to be provocative for the patient's symptoms, this is the segment and aspect that needs to be addressed in a grade-appropriate fashion; this is rarely the case in the pelvic pain population. If the clinician suspects a spinal segment involvement based upon the patient's history, clinical presentation, and special tests, the clinician is best served by applying a progressive posterior-to-anterior pressure using a split finger technique. With practice, patience, and a keen awareness of tissue reactivity, the clinician will notice that one side is typically more restrictive. This

restriction is commonly associated with a light fasciculation of the local musculature. Grade-appropriate mobilizations can then be administered along that aspect of that spinal segment for 60 to 90 seconds, and then the clinician can reassess one of the findings from the examination. A reduction in quality, intensity, and severity of symptoms indicates a successful examination, and treatment paradigm.[3,4,43]

Treatments should respect the findings of the stretch assessments. If the segment were found to be stiff, a mobilization of a grade III, IV, or V would be utilized (► Fig. 5.1), and if pain and protective muscle spasms were the primary findings, a grade I or II would be utilized. By definition, a grade I mobilization produces a small amplitude of motion within the first quarter of available motion. A grade II mobilization produces a greater amplitude that carries into the mid-range of available motion at that segment. A grade III produces greater amplitude of movement that extends into the fourth quarter, returning to the first quarter, shy of completely releasing the mobilization. A grade IV mobilization is a short amplitude oscillation within the last quarter of available segmental motion. A grade V mobilization is the spinal adjustment, or manipulation, which consists of a short-amplitude, high-velocity thrust that takes the tissue just beyond its anatomical limit.[43]

The clinician is to introduce a spinal mobilization when the pattern of pain reflects the potential for a segmental restriction. Reflecting upon the referral patterns from the zygoapophyseal joints, viscera, segmental distribution (dermatome), and the potential existence of extrasegmental references of pain, the clinician compares the patient's presenting findings and subsequently applies a segmental mobilization as a component of the evaluation. Regardless of symptom duration, the application of a spinal mobilization has been shown to impart a positive impact on the suffering patient's pain or muscle spasm. Prior to the application of a mobilization, the clinician is to pay close attention to the patient's surface anatomy to ensure an accurate segmental mobilization for the desired outcome.

There are two primary reasons that the spine will be addressed for the suffering patient: the patient has a stiff joint, arthrosis, which is referring pain, or the patient is demonstrating muscle spasms. As for the stiffened joint, the clinician is to impart a grade III or IV oscillatory mobilization, and if appropriate, a grade V. In the stiffest of joints, the clinician may consider utilizing an end-range, static mobilization. By slowly, comfortably loading the joint, creep deformation is allowed to occur, and hysteresis occurs.[78] In the treatment of pain and/or muscle spasm, the clinician best serves the patient by performing mobilizations in the grade I or II range of motion.

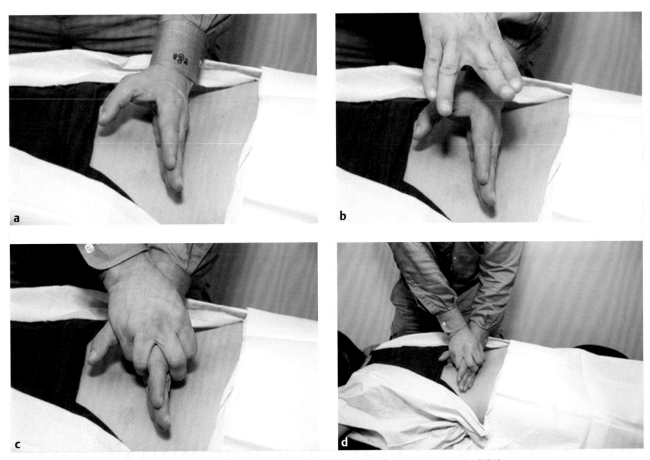

Fig. 5.2 a-d Mobilization hand positioning: central posterior-to-anterior (CPA)/unilateral posterior-to-anterior (UPA).

5.4.1 Rhythm

The use of staccato technique is in the treatment of a stiffened joint. It is performed to the joint's maximal range, but short of adjacent segment movement. With the minimally painful joint, the rhythm of the technique should be as if plucking a violin string. With a moderately painful joint, the speed of the technique should be more similar to staccato notes produced on a bow of a violin. With the painful joint, the oscillations are to be smooth and evenly transitioned from "on" to "off" so that the difference is difficult to discern.[43] For mobilization with CPA vertebral pressure the patient is prone on the plinth. The clinician positions him/herself over the segment to be treated, and applies a pressure through the fifth metacarpal on the spinous process in a gradual, progressive manner. Avoiding pisiform to the spinous process contact will assist with patient comfort. Throughout the application of a mobilization, the clinician's shoulders are to be positioned over the spinous process of the segment and the wrists are to be maintained in maximal extension, the forearm held midway between full supination and pronation. The mobilizing hand is to be reinforced by fitting the opposite hand over the mobilizing hand with a split finger technique. A mobilization utilizing unilateral posterior-anterior (UPA) vertebral pressure will be as that with CPA pressure with the exception that the contact and force transmission is through the respective transverse process.[43] The clinician is to keep in mind the that the transverse processes' of the thoracic spine are not necessarily adjacent to the vertebral body. Following the guidelines in the Clinical Note, the clinician is to use the width of the patient's finger when measuring distances; an approximation is taken with the width of the patient's index finger to that of the clinicians'.

> **Clinical Note**
>
> Thoracic spine palpation of transverse process rules:
>   T1 and T2: 1 patient finger width cranial to spinous process
>   T3 and T4: 2 patient fingers width cranial to spinous process
>   T5 to T8: 3 patient fingers width cranial to spinous process
>   T9 and T10: 2 patient fingers width cranial to spinous process

The technique of a CPA and a UPA mobilization is as follows (▶ Fig. 5.2). The clinician accurately palpates for the appropriate segment, placing the fatty portion of the hypothenar eminence on that spinous process or transverse process, as indicated by evaluation. A "knife-blade" technique is used with the web space between digit one and two being held in approximately 90 degrees of abduction. A split finger technique with the superior hand is then used to reinforce the knife-blade hand. The clinician's chest and sternum is to be positioned directly over the hands that are contacting the spine, and a progressive pressure is to be applied through the clinician's hands to the patient's spine. The clinician is to maintain straight arms as the weight of his or her body provides the mobilization.

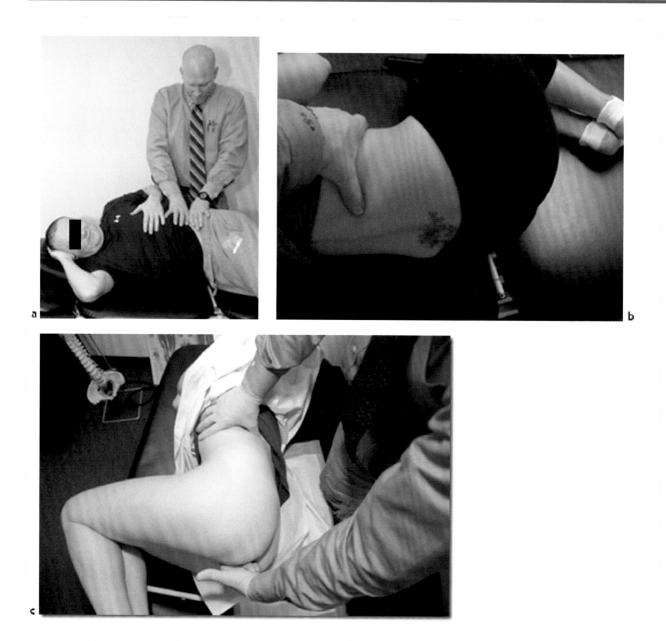

Fig. 5.3 a–c (a) Side-lying rotational mobilization with internal palpation. (b) Side-lying rotational mobilization technique. (c) Side-lying rotational mobilization set up.

5.4.2 Side-lying Rotational Mobilizations

The author has found the use of a side-lying, rotational mobilization to be quite effective in the elimination of pain, muscle spasm, and neurological entrapments. This technique, although simple in setup and execution, has demonstrated an efficiency and efficacy that is quite remarkable (▶ Fig. 5.3).

The patient is placed in the side-lying position with the painful side up. The patient's knees are taken in toward the chest, in hip flexion. The clinician takes his or her cranial hand and places the thumb in a fashion that is perpendicular to the patient's spine,

along the paraspinal mass. The caudal thumb reinforces the cranial thumb, and the clinician's sternum is held over the thumbs, with elbows straight. The mobilization is imparted through the muscle mass and directed at the lateral aspect of the spinous process, imparting a rotational mobilization.

5.4.3 Sacroiliac Joint Mobilization

During the course of the evaluation, if the clinician finds that the SIJ is unilaterally hypomobile, or there was positive pain provocation in testing, the clinician may consider utilizing the following SIJ mobilizations.

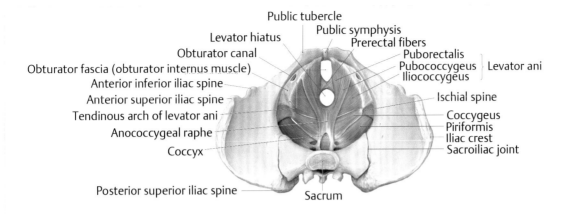

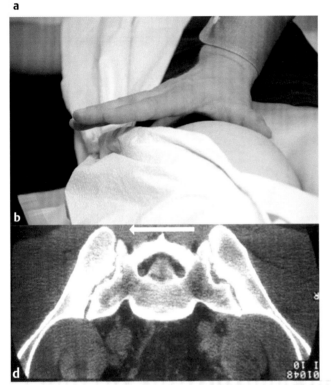

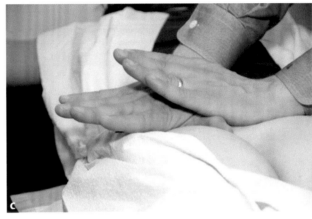

Fig. 5.4 a–d Local sacroiliac joint traction. ([a] from THIEME Atlas of Anatomy, General Anatomy and Musculoskeletal System, © Thieme 2005, illustration by Karl Wesker.)

Sacroiliac Joint Traction According to Grieve

With the patient prone on the plinth, knees off the edge, the clinician is to wrap a mobilization belt over the bent knee on the side of the hypomobile SIJ. The belt is then wrapped around the clinician's hips. The stabilization hand is placed, with permission, on the patient's sacral apex and a progressive traction is applied through the femur and coxofemoral joint to impart a mobilization force through the SIJ. This can be held, or oscillated as previously discussed in Section 5.4.1.[6]

Local sacroiliac joint traction

With the patient prone on the plinth and a pillow at the pelvis, the clinician places the cranial thumb along the medial border of the posterior iliac flare (▶ Fig. 5.4). The palpating digit is reinforced with the caudal hand, the heel of the hand. The mobilization is applied as a force that is parallel to the floor.

5.4.4 Sacral Thrust

With the patient prone, a CPA mobilization is applied to the spinous process of S4–5. The clinician's shoulders are maintained above the contact point, and the stretch articulation is noted, and the appropriate grade treatment is offered.

5.4.5 Sacral Mobilization with Movement

When the clinician finds that the sacrum is in a nutated position and is resistant to counternutationm then a mobilization with movement can be utilized. With the patient prone, and a pillow under her hip, the clinician aligns her sternum over the patient's sacrum, arms extended, and a hypothenar pressure is applied to the lower half of the sacrum. The patient is then asked to perform a contraction of her PFM, during which time the clinician assists in the movement of the sacrum into the counternutated position. After a 10-second hold, the patient relaxes and the clinician maintains the same pressure and alignment. This is repeated four times.

5.4.6 Massage/Transverse Friction Massage

Transverse friction massage (TFM) can be applied to both internal and external musculature. The application of TFM is intended to release adhesions found within a muscle belly, muscle-tendon junction, and/or the teno-periosteal junction. Due to excessive straining, sustained contractions, and/or local trauma, the muscle-tendon units can be partially torn, both microscopically and macroscopically. The local response is the laying down of scar or cross-adhesions across the sarcomeres, which in and of itself will act as an irritant to the adjacent musculotendinous structures based of their lack of pliability. The localized limitations of tissue mobility will initiate pain and decrease the immediately surrounding tissue to a taut state, impeding its local motion and leading to local scarring. Without direct treatment, a progression of scarring is common.[3,4]

A TFM is a massage that is performed in a rhythmical fashion perpendicular to the length of the muscle-tendon's fiber alignment. The application of a TFM should be comfortable and progressive, using firm pressure, without causing pain. As the body accommodates to the pressure, the clinician has the opportunity to increase the pressure as needed. The purpose of a TFM is to release adhesions, increase local circulation, and improve the proliferation of fibroblast development. The TFM can be applied to a ligament, muscle belly, muscle-tendon junction, and/or the teno-periosteal junction of both internal and external structures. As indicated by its name, the technique is performed by applying the massage force perpendicular to the orientation of the ligamentous, muscular, or tendinous fibers. In doing so, the clinician enhances tissue mobility, increasing the rate of phagocytosis and deposition of healing collagenous tissue by the removal of immature and weakened scar tissue, while promoting linear arrangement of bundles of connective tissue.

The trained clinician is able to discern normal tissue from tissue that is scarred. The term *crepitus* is used to describe the rough-and-course sensation under the clinician's palpating finger in regions of local scarring. When the clinician runs a finger over a region of crepitus, it will either be felt as "sand in a zipped storage bag" or as a "ridged potato chip in a zipped storage bag." The patient often expresses discomfort upon discovery of this lesion. The trained clinician is able to gently discern the presence of crepitus and often is able to locate the patient's pain source prior to the patient experiencing any pain. Thorough knowledge of the involved musculature is imperative to ensure that a proper technique is employed; as is evident, the internal musculature and ligaments are palpated and direct visualization is impossible. Depending upon the extent of crepitus noted, the treatment can last from 5 to 15 minutes.

The following is an explanation of how to directly impart a TFM to the pelvic structures. The clinician, with practice, can learn to discern the subtle changes in fiber alignment so as to best practice tissue-specific treatment.

Layer one structures of the pelvis:

Superficial transverse perineal

Location: From the ischial spine to the perineum
Technique: Physical therapist (PT) forearm resting on plinth. Digit-reinforced-digit (DRD) applied to region of crepitus; pronation and supination.

Ischiocavernosus

Location: Along ischium running midline and anterior
Technique: PT forearm resting on plinth, digit angled along ischium. DRD applied along region of crepitus.

Bulbocavernosus

Location: Midline from female (F) clitoral hood/male (M) corpus cavernosum and pubis
Technique: (F) pincer grasp between digit two and one. TFM imparted by wrist flexion and extension. (M) forearm resting on plinth. DRD applied to region of crepitus; pronation and supination.

Urethra

Location: Posterior to pubic symphasis
Technique: (F) PT forearm resting on plinth in full supination. Palpating digit maximally inserted and flexed maximally. TFM imparted by wrist flexion and extension. (M) PT forearm resting on plinth in full supination. Palpating digit maximally inserted and flexed maximally. TFM imparted by wrist flexion and extension. Care is to be taken due to the prostate.

Lower vagina

Location: Noted during vaginal sweep
Technique: PT forearm resting on plinth. The degree of pronation/supination is dependent upon location.

Labia minora/majora

Location: Noted during evaluation along length
Technique: Forearm neutral, gentle pincer grasp between digit one and two. TFM produced w/wrist flexion/extension.

Clitoral hood

Location: Noted during deflection during evaluation
Technique: Gentle pincer grasp between digit one and two. TFM produced w/ wrist flexion/extension.

Layer two structures of the pelvis:

Deep transverse perineal

Location: From both ischial spines to the perineum
Technique: Gentle pincer grasp between internal digit one and external digit two. Forearm in neutral alignment between pronation:supination. TFM produced with radial:ulnar deviation.

Compresser urethrae

Location: Anterior vagina; posterior to pubic symphysis; surrounding urethra
Technique: PT forearm resting on plinth in full supination. Palpating digit maximally inserted and flexed at metacarpal phalangeal (MCP) joint. TFM imparted with wrist flexion/extension.

Sphincter urethrae

Location: Circumferentially around urethra; posterior to pubic symphysis

Technique: PT forearm resting on plinth in full supination. Palpating digit maximally inserted and flexed at MCP. TFM imparted with wrist flexion/extension.

Layer three structures of pelvis:

Puborectalis (levator ani)

Location: Superior pubic rami to anococcygeal ligament

Technique: PT forearm resting on plinth. Digit applied to affected region. Superior aspect: forearm fully supinated; TFM imparted via radial:ulnar deviation. Middle aspect: forearm neutral and treating ipsilateral muscle; TFM imparted via wrist flexion/extension. Inferior/insertion: via rectum; forearm pronated; TFM via radial: ulnar deviation. Pubovaginalis/rectalis external reference point: Pubovaginalis, immediately lateral to the pubic symphysis; Puborectalis, ~1/4-1/2 of an inch lateral to the pubic symphysis.

Pubococcygeus (levator ani)

Location: Pubis, lateral to the puborectalis to the anococcygeal ligament

Technique: PT forearm resting on plinth; digit applied to affected region. Superior aspect: forearm fully supinated; TFM imparted via radial:ulnar deviation. Middle aspect: forearm neutral and treating ipsilateral muscle. TFM imparted via wrist flexion/extension. Inferior/insertion: via rectum; Forearm pronated; TFM imparted via radial: ulnar deviation. External reference point: just medial to the pubic tubercle.

Iliococcygeus

Location: Internal obturator fascia of levator ani to the anococcygeal ligament

Technique: PT forearm resting on plinth. Digit applied to affected region. Superior aspect: forearm fully supinated; TFM imparted via radial:ulnar deviation. Middle aspect: forearm neutral and treating ipsilateral muscle; TFM imparted via wrist flexion/extension. Inferior/insertion: via rectum; forearm pronated; TFM via radial:ulnar deviation.

Coccygeus

Location: Inferior apex of sacrum to the ischial spine

Technique: Rectal approach. PT forearm in full pronation. TFM imparted via wrist flexion/extension.

Obturator internus

Location: Obturator membrane and bony boundaries of obturator foramen to the greater trochanter of the femur

Technique: PT forearm resting on plinth in neutral alignment. TFM imparted via pronation:supination.

Anterior SIJ ligament

Location: Traversing the length of the anterior SIJ

Technique: PT forearm in neutral alignment and angled 45 degrees in posterior, cranial fashion. TFM imparted via radial: ulnar deviation. (Note: patient's knees/hips may be flexed to allow appropriate access to ligament.)

Posterior ligaments of the SIJ:

Sacrotuberous

Location: Along SIJ posteriorly from posterior superior iliac spine (PSIS) and lateral sacrum/coccyx to the ischial tuberosity

Technique: PT places cranial thumb along SIJ, standing contralateral to the side being addressed. This palpating digit is reinforced with contralateral thumb or heel of hand. TFM imparted via protraction:retraction of scapula for vertical fibers, and via trunk side flexion for horizontal fibers.

Iliolumbar ligament

Location: Approximately 1 inch superior and lateral to PSIS, along anterior ilium

Technique: PT stands on contralateral to the side being addressed, cranially. PT presses along iliac crest in posterior-anterior-lateral fashion with DRD. TFM imparted via protraction:retraction of shoulder.

Interosseus ligament

Location: Anterior and superior to PSIS, deep within sulcus between iliac crest and sacrum

Technique: PT stands contralateral to side being addressed. DRD applied to sulcus. TFM imparted via pronation:supination.

Long posterior SIJ ligament

Location: Along the sacral spinous processes to posterior flare of ilium

Technique: PT stands contralateral to side being addressed. Cranial thumb is laid along the lateral border of spinous processes with angulation in superior-lateral fashion toward flare of ilium. TFM imparted via side flexion of trunk.

Sacrospinous ligament

Location: Along sacrococcygeal junction to the iliac spine

External: PT stands ipsilateral to side being addressed. PT palpates lateral to the sacrococcygeal joint, pressing firmly in posterior-to-anterior fashion, and then cranially to address inferior aspect of ligament. TFM imparted via shoulder protraction:retraction.

Internal: PT is supine in lithotomy position. PT with forearm on plinth, in full pronation. Rectal approach and TFM imparted via wrist Flexion/extension.

A "milking" technique can be utilized if the TFM is found to be too painful. This involves the use of a massaging pincer grasp that runs parallel to the fibers of the muscle-tendon unit in an attempt to increase local circulation. Gliding over the tender spot may induce discomfort, so care is to be taken.

In the presence of local scars, internally or externally, the clinician must maximally restore tissue pliability. This not only restores functional, interactive mobility of the local structures, but also reduces itching, eases distress, reduces pain and anxiety, and generally improves mood. Depending on location, scars can also limit range of motion of underlying joints.[79,80]

Cutaneous scar management can begin as soon as a wound has healed.[81] All massage techniques should be firm enough to make the skin blanch, the pressure should build up gradually as blistering may occur. The typical massage is performed in a circular fashion, and the patient can be taught to do this independently.[82] It is believed that massage breaks up collagen fibers, despite little supportive evidence.[79,81,82] Suffice to say, if scars are present and confounding, they are to be addressed directly. Utilizing the techniques outlined below, a slow, progressive treatment approach will assist in the restoration of fascial mobility and further assist in the healing process.

Both internal and external scars along the dermis will respond well to circular massage. The clinician, using a DRD technique, locates the scar and then applies a firm but not hard pressure into the tissue so as to establish a connection between the DRD and the scarred dermis. The movement of the DRD is to carry the scarred dermis versus sliding over the scarred dermis. The pressure should be light at first, allowing accommodation to occur, and gently progressing in pressure to further engage the scarred tissue. This should never be painful, but it will be felt by the patient. Internal scars require a keen awareness of the local anatomy, in particular that which are the normal ridges (rugae) of the vagina. A scar will feel like a ridge that is more firm to palpation and will demonstrate restrictions in mobility. Pain may be noted by the patient with palpation of a scar, but not necessarily; neurological accommodation can be quite deceiving. The massage should last for 5 to 15 minutes. Immediate changes in tissue texture are to be expected.

Definitive benefits of massage on scars are difficult to find in the literature. Reported, short-term benefits include: enhanced trust between the patient and clinician, improved skin quality, relieved sensitivity, increased cutaneous hydration, improved scar quality, better acceptance of the lesion by patient, reduction of patient's anxiety, and enhancement of mood and mental status.[79,81] In the evaluation of the patient with pelvic pain, scars should be evaluated for and treated where restrictions are present. This is inclusive of scars along the abdomen, external hip, saddle region, and intravaginal and rectal regions. When compared with superficial touch/massage, deep tissue massage was shown to be able to reduce mechanical hyperalgesia and stretch pain.[83] Long-term benefits associated with scar massage have been noted and have been seen as a reduction of depression, anger, and decreased pain as measured by the McGill Pain Questionnaire, present pain intensity scale, and visual analog scale.[79] Massage-like stimulation in rats has shown an increase in the endogenous release of oxytocin in plasma and PAG, and the antinociceptive effects are prevented by blockade of oxytocin receptors. Oxytocin is a hormone that is shown to increase pain threshold, inducing physical relaxation, and to lower blood pressure and cortisol levels. It therefore is speculated that massage may decrease hyperalgesia and pain through activation of descending inhibitory pathways using the PAG-opioid system and oxytocin.[83]

Skin rolling and scar rolling is another form of massage that is beneficial in the restoration of appropriate connective tissue mobility. Whether rolling across skin or scar, the technique is the same; a pinch of skin is taken and "rolled" into the direction of limitation or restriction. In regions of severe restrictions, an audible "click" may be noted, but is not necessary for healing. (Clinical side note: Along the thoracolumbosacral fascia, the absence of restrictions and audible release will indicate to the clinician patient compliance with the maintenance of neutral posture as the relative joints will be under less irritation and

inflammation and the fascia will maintain appropriate length tension.) Scars, old and new, respond well to skin rolling[84] and both clinician and patient alike are often wonderfully surprised as to a newfound wellness after the provision of a scar massage.

A trigger point is a painful muscle nodule, which gives rise to a palpable fasciculation upon strumming, and produces a distinct and predictable referral pattern; each muscle has a unique referral pattern.[85] All painful muscle nodules are not trigger points; in fact, the majority are muscle tender points. The differentiation is important for both clinician and patient. Massaging, ischemic pressures, and "press-and-stretch" to a tender point will *not* have long-lasting benefit for the patient. Tender points, however, will rapidly respond and be eliminated with an appropriate joint mobilization. Knowing which joint to mobilize requires the clinician to have a firm grasp on embryology as it relates to somatically related structures, and a keen sense of appropriate arthrokinematic motions. Determining the cause of the tender spot within the muscle is imperative, and direct treatment thereto will offer the patient immediate relief of pain and the tender spot will "release" immediately.

There are many examples of the presence of local muscle tender spots that are *not* trigger points. One of the most common is the upper trapezius tension/muscle spasm that is common among the general population. These tender spots are often the result of inflammation and restrictions at the sternoclavicular joint (SCJ) and the all too common "tight shoulder" will experience complete relaxation and release of "spasm" after the application of a grade I to II oscillatory mobilization to the SCJ, and or the application of ice to the SCJ.[3] If there were a true lesion of the upper trapezius, or the pain were due to an intrinsic injury to the upper trapezius, then the application of a mobilization or ice to the SCJ would have no impact on this structure. To the great surprise of many clinicians and patients alike, this treatment works exceptionally well; this concept can be applied throughout the body. Other common examples are "piriformis syndrome," which responds well to L1–2 UPA mobilizations, and iliopsoas tender spots, which respond well to T12 to L1 UPA mobilizations.[86]

If, after each structure and joint that can refer to a particular region has been exhaustively evaluated, and the clinician has applied appropriate motion, a tender spot within a muscle persists, and if it has the characteristic "twitch" with strumming and gives rise to a pre-determined referred pain pattern, then it may be considered a trigger point. The current understanding is that a trigger point will compress the local sensory nerve inducing a reduction of axoplasmic transport of molecules that normally inhibit acetylcholine (Ach) release, while also compressing the local blood vessels resulting in a local ischemic event. This further depletes the adenosine triphosphate (ATP) concentration. The result is an ATP energy crisis that triggers a cascade of pre/postsynaptic decompensations. Postsynaptically speaking, ATP powers the calcium pump that returns calcium to the sarcoplasmic reticulum. ATP directly inhibits Ach release presynaptically; a depletion of ATP effectively will increase the Ach release, resulting in increased contractile activity and a self-perpetuating cycle, an "ATP energy crisis."[2]

As Langford et al found, trigger point injection was effective at decreasing local muscle spasm when there was a highly selective group of patients seeking treatment of "levator ani syndrome." Their study demonstrated a 72.2% improvement of status after the first injection.[87] In the 1999 edition of *Myofascial Pain and Dysfunction: The Trigger Point Manual*, the editors abandoned the application of a heavy, ischemic compression for the treatment of trigger points.[85] In its place, they proposed a novel trigger point release technique that they referred to as "press-and-stretch." This technique is applied with a single finger palpating the affected muscle band. When a trigger point is encountered, the clinician passively lengthens it to the point of tissue resistance. This engaged barrier is held until a release is palpated. The clinician then "follows" the release until a second barrier is noted. This process is repeated until there are no further barriers to be found within the affected muscle. The hypothesis is that the technique mechanically uncouples the myosin from actin in an attempt to short circuit the "energy crisis cycle."[2]

5.5 Exercise Concepts

The gradual introduction of exercises that address the individual's postural faults is necessary to ensure the patient's complete healing, and to further assess the patient's willingness to be an active participant in her healing process. The exercises are to be gentle enough so they do not aggravate the prevailing pain condition, and yet specific enough to promote healing. It is often a fine line that the clinician must walk with his or her pelvic pain patients; reconditioning without "straining" is the goal. Attached are samples of exercises that may be used to address a patient's de-conditioned state, but are not to be considered

exclusive. As the patient progresses with her reconditioning, more dynamic exercises can be introduced that more readily replicate the common stresses the patient will experience throughout the day.

A common starting point for the patient recovering from a pelvic pain is to ensure proper isolation of the PFM. To best accomplish this, the clinician utilizes a split finger technique as outlined in Chapter 3. The patient is to be encouraged to utilize the PFM in isolation of accessory musculature contraction: gluteals, respiration holding, hip adductors, or other. The clinician is to ensure that the patient is coordinating each layer of the pelvic floor, progressing from the first layer to the third. Stretch facilitation is often required where weaknesses present themselves, often unilaterally.

Once the patient can isolate the PFM, diaphragmatic respiration is to be introduced while the patient maintains an appropriate PFM contraction. The clinician is often required to provide facilitation via rapid, gentle outward digital pressures, when the patient loses contraction. Often the coordination of the PFM with activity is quite a difficult task for the patient.

As the patient's capacity and confidence improves, the clinician will progress the patient's reconditioning exercises to include the integration of more challenging maneuvers such as the "bridge," where the patient is asked to raise the pelvis from the treatment table, hold for a set time, and then lower back to the table, all while maintaining the PFM contraction (▶ Fig. 5.5). Again, the clinician will do well to palpate the PFM during and throughout the performance of the "bridge."

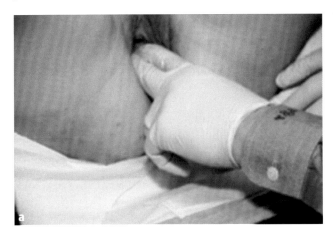
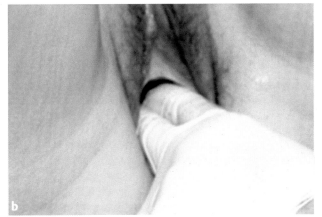
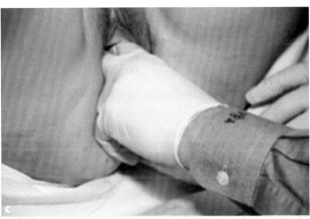

Fig. 5.5 a–c Split finger assessment of the pelvic floor musculature: layers one, two, and three.

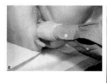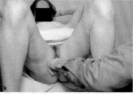

Fig. 5.6 a,b Pelvic floor contraction during abdominal crunches.

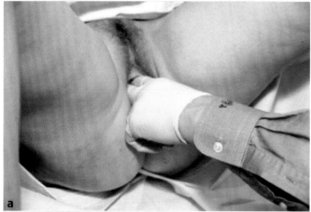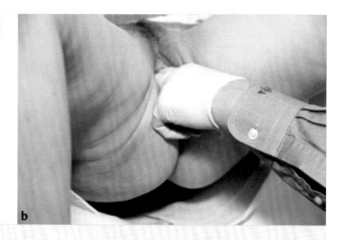

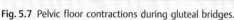

Fig. 5.7 Pelvic floor contractions during gluteal bridges.

This concept can be applied to the performance of an abdominal crunch and other open kinetic chain and closed kinetic chain exercises alike. The most challenging for the patient is the performance of a free-standing squat while maintaining PFM contractions throughout the available range of motion (▶ Fig. 5.8). During the introduction of the palpating digit(s) during a standing exercise with internal palpation, it is suggested that the clinician have the patient assist in the introduction of the palapting digit so as not to compromise hygiene by inadvertently contacting the anus. Once the palpating digit(s) have been placed, the patient is asked to engage the PFM, and then while maintaining the contraction, perform a free-standing squat. If and when the contraction is lost, a verbal cue or quick-stretch facilitation may be useful at re-engaging the PFM. The patient may only be capable of maintaining the PFM contraction in a limited range of motion; that's OK. As the patient increases their awareness and strength, they will demonstrate increased capacity to maintain the contraction of the PFM through greater and greater degrees of motion. With the patient suffering from a pelvic prolapse, she may be taught to self reduce by using a rhythmic contraction of the pelvic layers one, two, and three. By sequencing her contractions, she may be able to not only reduce the prolapse, but maintain the reduction independently. The utilization of a manual lift, by herself or with assistance of the clinician, may be required in order to allow the musculature to contract, as the musculature itself is often inhibited in the presence of a descending viscus.

The following exercises are to be considered in the treatment of our patients with pelvic pain and dysfunction. All choices of exercises should be made on a patient-to-patient basis as appropriate. It is recommended that the following verbal

cuing be used for appropriate activation of the pelvic floor musculature:
- Layer One: "Pinch"
- Layer Two: "Squeeze"
- Layer Three: "Embrace then Lift"

This terminology allows for the patient to readily appreciate the major role each muscle layer has, while also encouraging appropriate sequencing and activation of the pelvic floor. Doing so will provide the following:
- Improved visceral stability; many patients can be taught how to self-reduce minor prolapses
- Improved spinal stability
- Enhanced orgasms

Each layer and each side of the vagina can be encouraged to exercise both the fast-twitch and the slow-twitch musculature. Common practice includes having the patient work up to 100 consecutive fast twitch contractions, and 10 10-second contractions.

In the presence of a prolapse, the clinician can provide the appropriate lift to the descending structure and educate the patient to perform the aforementioned contractions below the viscus so as to allow for better muscle activation and reduction of prolapse (▶ Fig. 5.5).

Resisted range of motion to the pelvic floor musculature is an efficient means to enhance coordination and strength of a weakened layer, or local within the pelvic floor musculature. The weaknesses may be due to traumatic scarring from birthing or otherwise, myopathic lesions, or generalized weakness. The

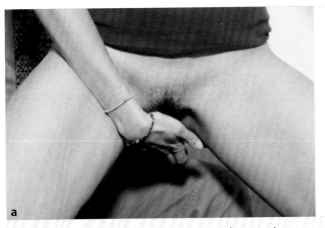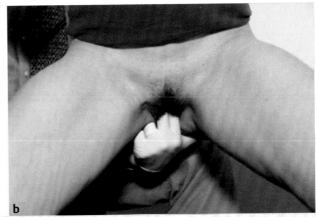

Fig. 5.8 Pelvic floor contractions during squatting, lunges and yoga.

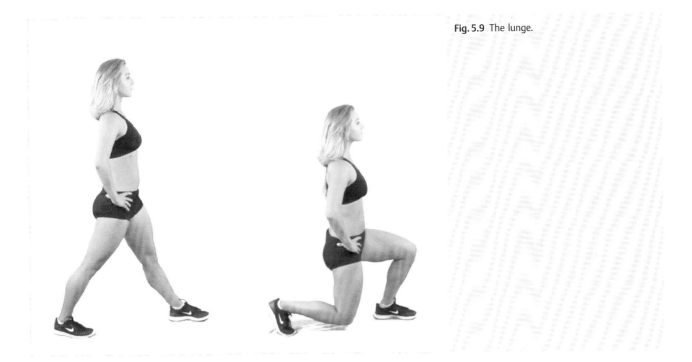

Fig. 5.9 The lunge.

technique is applied with a single digit or dual digit as appropriate, and the patient is encouraged to perform a contraction at the desired layer, or coordinate the three layers. A quick stretch often provides the feedback required to initiate a weakened section of musculature.

Encouraging and monitoring appropriate pelvic floor muscle contractions during therapeutic exercises have proven themselves to be quite effective as a tool in enhancing a patient's recovery, and long term success. The performance of an internal palpation of the pelvic floor can be used in most any exercise, and below are the most common utilized.

Pelvic floor contraction during abdominal crunches (▶ Fig. 5.8):

The clinician is to comfortably insert a single or double digit as appropriate for each patient. The clinician is to instruct the patient to perform a sequential contraction from level one, level two, and finally level three musculature, and is asked to maintain this throughout the exercise. A bridge is then performed as the clinician monitors the patient's capacity to maintain continual contractions throughout. Often it is required that a verbal, or tactile cuing be offered to encourage continued pelvic floor contractions throughout the movement.

Pelvic floor contractions during squatting, lunges and yoga (▶ Fig. 5.9):

This maneuver has proven itself to be very effective in providing functional stability of the pelvis, sacroiliac joint, and lumbar spine. Many patients and clinicians alike are taken aback at just how difficult it is to perform and maintain a pelvic floor muscle contraction throughout weight-bearing, dynamic activities and exercises. It is recommended that the patient be allowed to insert the clinician's digit(s) themselves so as to avoid unintended contact with the anus. While in the starting

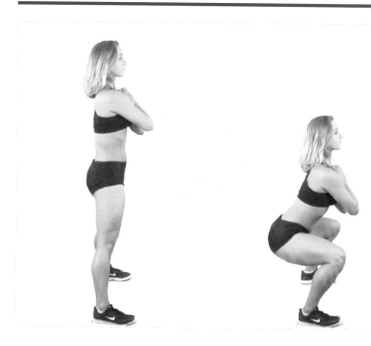

Fig. 5.10 The squat.

position the patient is encouraged to perform a sequential contraction from level one, level two, and finally level three musculature, and is asked to maintain this throughout the exercise. The patient then performs a squat, lunge, yoga pose, or that activity where they are having difficulty stabilizing their pelvis, pelvic floor, sacroiliac joint, or lumbar spine.

The following exercises can be used to encourage appropriate pelvic stability, with or without internal palpation.

The lunge (▶ Fig. 5.9):
- Stand in a stride position with one foot behind you, on the toes
- Keep the ear, shoulder, and hip in one line as you bring your left knee towards the floor
- Keep the pelvic and abdominal muscles held tight
  ○ Never strike the knee to the floor
- Repeat 10–30 times as recommended
  ○ Repeat with your opposite foot behind you
- Additional difficulty:
  ○ Hold at the lowest angle/depth of lunge for 2/5/7/10 seconds
  ○ Raise 3/4s up, and then lower
  ○ Repeat

The squat (▶ Fig. 5.10):
- Stand with feet more than shoulders width apart and the toes pointed out ten degrees
- Roll the hips backward, as if you were sitting in a chair, while keeping your pelvic and abdominal muscle contracted
- The arms are held across your chest as the trunk is taken into a forward lean 20 degrees
  ○ Bend both knees to comfort
  ○ Keep the pressure through your heels
- Repeat 10–30 times as recommended

- Additional difficulty:
  ○ Hold at the lowest angle/depth of squat for 2/5/7/10 seconds
  ○ Raise 3/4s up, and then lower
  ○ Repeat

Unilateral standing with knee flexion (▶ Fig. 5.11):
- Stand on one foot
- Contract the pelvic floor musculature, abdominals, and gluteals
- Do not lean to the side
- While keeping your knees parallel, flex the nonstanding knee
- Hold for 3/5/10 seconds, and repeat 10/20/30 times

Unilateral standing with hip abduction (▶ Fig. 5.12):
- Stand on one foot
- Contract the pelvic floor musculature, abdominals, and gluteals
- While keeping erect, raise one foot to the side; do not lean
- Hold for 3/5/10 seconds, and repeat 10/20/30 times

Standard abdominals (▶ Fig. 5.13):
- While supine with knees bent/feet flat, the hands are to be placed under head/neck
  ○ Keep the chin tucked in as the head and chest are raised toward the ceiling (not towards the knees)
  ○ Hold for 3/5/10 seconds, repeat 20/15/10x

Oblique abdominals (▶ Fig. 5.14):
- While supine, place hands under head/neck
- Rotate your knees to the left 45 degrees left

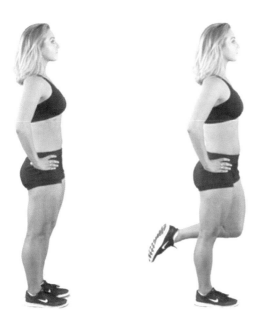

Fig. 5.11 Unilateral standing with knee flexion.

Fig. 5.12 Unilateral standing with hip abduction.

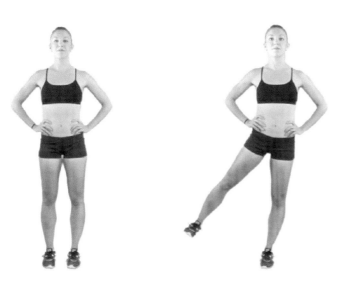

- Keep the chin tucked in as the head and chest are raised toward the ceiling
  - Once at the uppermost of motion, twist to the right
  - Maintain the twist and elevate towards the ceiling a little more
  - Hold for 3/5/10 seconds lower your right shoulder toward the floor, all whilst maintaining the rotation
  - Repeat 20/15/10x
  - Repeat on the opposite side

Abdominal bridge with twist (▸ Fig. 5.15):
- Lie on the right side, resting on the right elbow/forearm
  - Keep the elbow directly under the shoulder so that the elbow is perpendicular to the floor and your top hand is on your head, elbow to ceiling.
- The body is held straight as the right hip is raised from the floor
  - Keep the right foot and right elbow/forearm on the floor
- At the apex of motion, twist the left shoulder toward the floor
  - Do not allow the hip/pelvis to sway or rotate

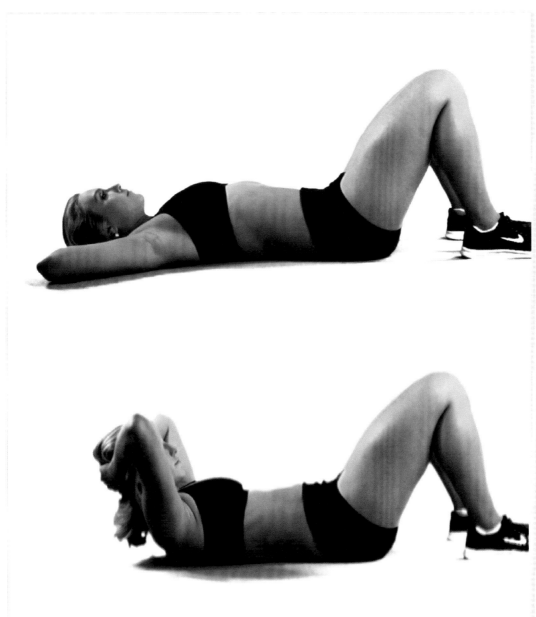

Fig. 5.13 Standard abdominals.

- Repeat 10–30 repetitions
- Repeat on the left side

Abdominal press (▶ Fig. 5.16):
- Lie on one side, hand supporting your head, opposite hand on the floor.
- Keep the top hip forward 10 degrees.
- Press through left hand and raise your right shoulder and head.
- Keep the body's orientation perpendicular to the floor.
- Hold for 3 seconds, and do 10–30 repetitions.
- Repeat on the opposite side.

Abdominal float (▶ Fig. 5.17):
- Lie on your side, head supported by left hand.
- Right hand is on the table in front of the chest for support.
  - Keep the top hip forward 10 degrees.
- Keeping the legs straight, and your left hip to the floor, elevate the legs together towards the ceiling.
  - Keep the body's orientation 10 degrees forward of perpendicular to the floor.
- Hold for 3 seconds, and repeat 10–30 repetitions.
- Repeat on the opposite side.

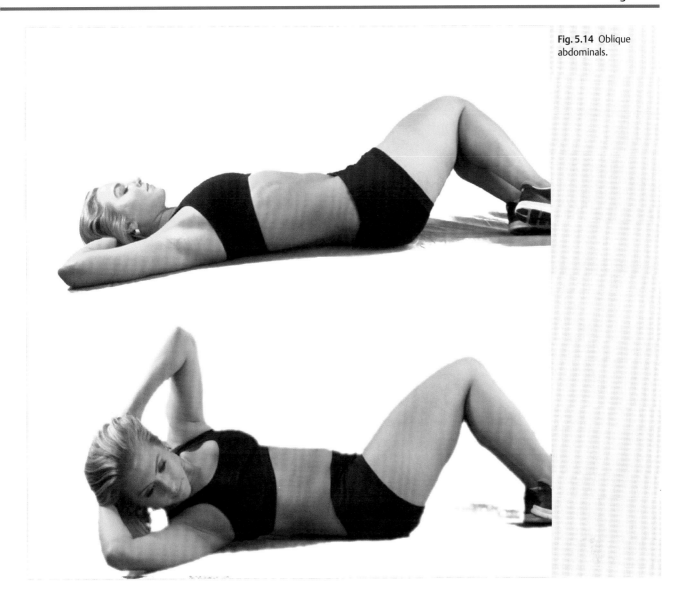

Fig. 5.14 Oblique abdominals.

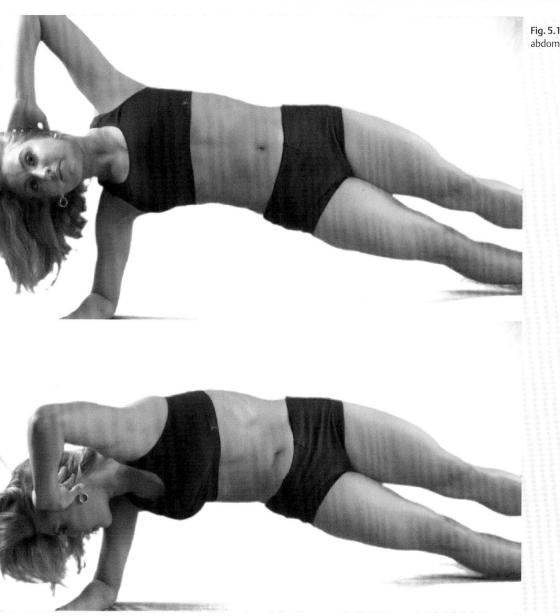

Fig. 5.15 Oblique abdominals.

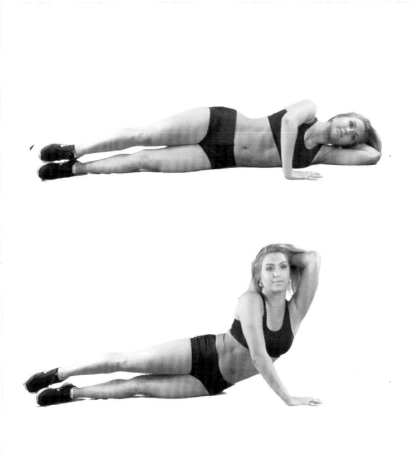

Fig. 5.16 Abdominal press.

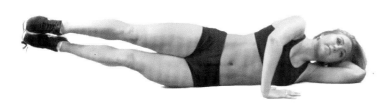

Fig. 5.17 Abdominal float.

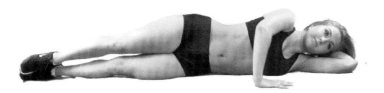

References

[1] Weström LV, Willén R. Vestibular nerve fiber proliferation in vulvar vestibulitis syndrome. Obstet Gynecol 1998; 91: 572–576

[2] McPartland JM. Travell trigger points—molecular and osteopathic perspectives. J Am Osteopath Assoc 2004; 104: 244–249

[3] Cyriax J, Ed. (1982). Textbook of orthopaedic medicine. London, Philadelphia, Toronto, Sydney & Tokyo: WB Saunders & Bailliere Tindall

[4] Ombregt L, Ed. (2003). A system of orthopaedic medicine (2nd ed.). Philadelphia, London: Churchill Livingstone

[5] Suni J, Rinne M, Natri A et al. Control of the lumbar neutral zone decreases low back pain and improves self-evaluated work ability: a 12-month randomized controlled study. Spine 2006; 31: E611–620

[6] Boyling JD, Ed. (2004). Grieve's modern manual therapy (3rd ed.). Edinburgh, London, New York, Oxford, Philadelphia, St. Louis, Sydney, Toronto: Churchill Livingstone

[7] Greenman PE, Ed. (1996). Principles of manual medicine (4th ed.) Lippincott Williams & Wilkins

[8] Howard FM, Ed. (2000). Pelvic pain: Diagnosis & management. Philadelphia, Baltimore, New York, London, Buenos Aires, Hong Kong, Sydney & Tokyo: Lippincott Williams & Wilkins

[9] Won HR, Abbott J. Optimal management of chronic cyclical pelvic pain: an evidence-based and pragmatic approach. Int J Womens Health 2010; 2: 263–277

[10] Harrison DD, Harrison SO, Croft AC, Harrison DE, Troyanovich SJ. Sitting biomechanics part I: review of the literature. J Manipulative Physiol Ther 1999; 22: 594–609

[11] Harrison DD, Harrison SO, Croft AC, Harrison DE, Troyanovich SJ. Sitting biomechanics, part II: optimal car driver's seat and optimal driver's spinal model. J Manipulative Physiol Ther 2000; 23: 37–47

[12] Harrison DE, Harrison DD, Troyanovich SJ. The sacroiliac joint: a review of anatomy and biomechanics with clinical implications. J Manipulative Physiol Ther 1997; 20: 607–617

[13] Harrison DE, Cailliet R, Harrison DD, Troyanovich SJ, Harrison SO. A review of biomechanics of the central nervous system—Part I: spinal canal deformations resulting from changes in posture. J Manipulative Physiol Ther 1999; 22: 227–234

[14] Harrison DE, Cailliet R, Harrison DD, Troyanovich SJ, Harrison SO. A review of biomechanics of the central nervous system—part II: spinal cord strains from postural loads. J Manipulative Physiol Ther 1999; 22: 322–332

[15] Harrison DE, Cailliet R, Harrison DD, Troyanovich SJ, Harrison SO. A review of biomechanics of the central nervous system—Part III: spinal cord stresses from postural loads and their neurologic effects. J Manipulative Physiol Ther 1999; 22: 399–410

[16] Harrison DE, Harrison DD, Harrison SO, Troyanovich SJ. A review of biomechanics of the central nervous system. Part 1: Spinal canal deformations caused by changes in posture. J Manipulative Physiol Ther 2000; 23: 217–220

[17] Hartmann D, Strauhal MJ, Nelson CA. Treatment of women in the United States with localized, provoked vulvodynia: practice survey of women's health physical therapists. J Reprod Med 2007; 52: 48–52

[18] Harris-Love MO, Shrader JA. Physiotherapy management of patients with HIV-associated Kaposi's sarcoma. Physiother Res Int 2004; 9: 174–181

[19] Williams RE, Black CL, Kim HY et al. Determinants of healthcare-seeking behaviour among subjects with irritable bowel syndrome. Aliment Pharmacol Ther 2006; 23: 1667–1675

[20] ter Kuile MM, Weijenborg PT, Spinhoven P. Sexual functioning in women with chronic pelvic pain: the role of anxiety and depression. J Sex Med 2010; 7: 1901–1910

[21] Ren K, Dubner R. Central nervous system plasticity and persistent pain. J Orofac Pain 1999; 13: 155–163, discussion 164–171

[22] Ren K, Dubner R. Inflammatory models of pain and hyperalgesia. ILAR Journal / National Research Council Institute of Laboratory Animal Resources 1999; 40: 111–118

[23] Pukall CF, Binik YM, Khalifé S, Amsel R, Abbott FV. Vestibular tactile and pain thresholds in women with vulvar vestibulitis syndrome. Pain 2002; 96: 163–175

[24] Ventegodt S, Thegler S, Andreasen T et al. Clinical holistic medicine: psychodynamic short-time therapy complemented with bodywork. A clinical follow-up study of 109 patients. ScientificWorldJournal 2006; 6: 2220–2238

[25] Sambajon VV, Cillo JE, Jr, Gassner RJ, Buckley MJ. The effects of mechanical strain on synovial fibroblasts. J Oral Maxillofac Surg 2003; 61: 707–712

[26] So C. How manipulation works. The Journal of the Hong Kong Physiotherapy Association 1986; 8: 30–34

[27] Cottingham JT, Porges SW, Lyon T. Effects of soft tissue mobilization (Rolfing pelvic lift) on parasympathetic tone in two age groups. Phys Ther 1988; 68: 352–356

[28] Cottingham JT, Maitland J. A three-paradigm treatment model using soft tissue mobilization and guided movement-awareness techniques for a patient with chronic low back pain: a case study. J Orthop Sports Phys Ther 1997; 26: 155–167

[29] Hurwitz EL, Aker PD, Adams AH, Meeker WC, Shekelle PG. Manipulation and mobilization of the cervical spine. A systematic review of the literature. Spine 1996; 21: 1746–1759, discussion 1759–1760

[30] Hurwitz EL, Morgenstern H, Harber P, Kominski GF, Yu F, Adams AH. A randomized trial of chiropractic manipulation and mobilization for patients with neck pain: clinical outcomes from the UCLA neck-pain study. Am J Public Health 2002; 92: 1634–1641

[31] Keller TS, Colloca CJ, Béliveau JG. Force-deformation response of the lumbar spine: a sagittal plane model of posteroanterior manipulation and mobilization. Clin Biomech (Bristol, Avon) 2002; 17: 185–196

[32] Jamison JR, McEwen AP, Thomas SJ. Chiropractic adjustment in the management of visceral conditions: a critical appraisal. J Manipulative Physiol Ther 1992; 15: 171–180

[33] Browning JE. Pelvic pain and organic dysfunction in a patient with low back pain: response to distractive manipulation: a case presentation. J Manipulative Physiol Ther 1987; 10: 116–121

[34] Weiss JM. Pelvic floor myofascial trigger points: manual therapy for interstitial cystitis and the urgency-frequency syndrome. J Urol 2001; 166: 2226–2231

[35] Allison G, Edmonston S, Kiviniemi K, Lanigan H, Simonsen AV, Walcher S. Influence of standardized mobilization on the posteroanterior stiffness of the lumbar spine in asymptomatic subjects. Physiother Res Int 2001; 6: 145–156

[36] Allison G. Effect of direction of applied mobilization force on the posteroanterior response in the lumbar spine. J Manipulative Physiol Ther 2001; 24: 487–488

[37] Dishman JD, Bulbulian R. Spinal reflex attenuation associated with spinal manipulation. Spine 2000; 25: 2519–2524, discussion 2525

[38] Dishman JD, Bulbulian R. Comparison of effects of spinal manipulation and massage on motoneuron excitability. Electromyogr Clin Neurophysiol 2001; 41: 97–106

[39] Dishman JD, Ball KA, Burke J. First Prize: central motor excitability changes after spinal manipulation: a transcranial magnetic stimulation study. J Manipulative Physiol Ther 2002; 25: 1–9

[40] Dishman JD, Cunningham BM, Burke J. Comparison of tibial nerve H-reflex excitability after cervical and lumbar spine manipulation. J Manipulative Physiol Ther 2002; 25: 318–325

[41] Dishman JD, Burke J. Spinal reflex excitability changes after cervical and lumbar spinal manipulation: a comparative study. Spine J 2003; 3: 204–212

[42] Oliphant D. Safety of spinal manipulation in the treatment of lumbar disk herniations: a systematic review and risk assessment. J Manipulative Physiol Ther 2004; 27: 197–210

[43] Maitland G, Ed. Maitland's vertebral manipulation. Edinburgh, London, New York, Oxford, Philadelphia, St. Louis, Sydney, Toronto: Elsevier; 2005

[44] Cascioli V, Corr P, Till Ag AG. An investigation into the production of intra-articular gas bubbles and increase in joint space in the zygapophyseal joints of the cervical spine in asymptomatic subjects after spinal manipulation. J Manipulative Physiol Ther 2003; 26: 356–364

[45] Wilson DG. Results of manipulation in general practice. Proc R Soc Med 1967; 60: 971–972

[46] Lehman GJ, McGill SM. The influence of a chiropractic manipulation on lumbar kinematics and electromyography during simple and complex tasks: a case study. J Manipulative Physiol Ther 1999; 22: 576–581

[47] Lehman GJ, McGill SM. Spinal manipulation causes variable spine kinematic and trunk muscle electromyographic responses. Clin Biomech (Bristol, Avon) 2001; 16: 293–299

[48] Lehman GJ, Vernon H, McGill SM. Effects of a mechanical pain stimulus on erector spinae activity before and after a spinal manipulation in patients with back pain: a preliminary investigation. J Manipulative Physiol Ther 2001; 24: 402–406

[49] Cramer GD, Ross K, Pocius J et al. Evaluating the relationship among cavitation, zygapophyseal joint gapping, and spinal manipulation: an exploratory case series. J Manipulative Physiol Ther 2011; 34: 2–14

[50] Lehto M, Järvinen M. Collagen and glycosaminoglycan synthesis of injured gastrocnemius muscle in rat. Eur Surg Res 1985; 17: 179–185

[51] Lehto M, Duance VC, Restall D. Collagen and fibronectin in a healing skeletal muscle injury. An immunohistological study of the effects of physical activity on the repair of injured gastrocnemius muscle in the rat. J Bone Joint Surg Br 1985; 67: 820–828

[52] George SZ, Bishop MD, Bialosky JE, Zeppieri G, Jr, Robinson ME. Immediate effects of spinal manipulation on thermal pain sensitivity: an experimental study. BMC Musculoskelet Disord 2006; 7: 68

[53] Jull GA, Falla D, Vicenzino B, Hodges PW. The effect of therapeutic exercise on activation of the deep cervical flexor muscles in people with chronic neck pain. Man Ther 2009; 14: 696–701

[54] Sluka KA. Pain mechanisms involved in musculoskeletal disorders. J Orthop Sports Phys Ther 1996; 24: 240–254

[55] Sluka KA, Christy MR, Peterson WL, Rudd SL, Troy SM. Reduction of pain-related behaviors with either cold or heat treatment in an animal model of acute arthritis. Arch Phys Med Rehabil 1999; 80: 313–317

[56] Sluka KA, Rohlwing JJ, Bussey RA, Eikenberry SA, Wilken JM. Chronic muscle pain induced by repeated acid injection is reversed by spinally administered mu- and delta-, but not kappa-, opioid receptor agonists. J Pharmacol Exp Ther 2002; 302: 1146–1150

[57] Song XJ, Gan Q, Cao JL, Wang ZB, Rupert RL. Spinal manipulation reduces pain and hyperalgesia after lumbar intervertebral foramen inflammation in the rat. J Manipulative Physiol Ther 2006; 29: 5–13

[58] Moore KL, Dalley AF, Eds. (2006). Clinically orientated anatomy (5th ed.). Baltimore, Philadelphia: Lippincott Williams & Wilkins

[59] Sluka KA, Skyba DA, Radhakrishnan R et al. Joint mobilization reduces hyperalgesia associated with chronic muscle and joint inflammation in rats. J Pain 2006; 7: 602–607

[60] Dishman JD, Dougherty PE, Burke JR. Evaluation of the effect of postural perturbation on motoneuronal activity following various methods of lumbar spinal manipulation. Spine J 2005; 5: 650–659

[61] Bittar P, Muller D. Time-dependent reversal of long-term potentiation by brief cooling shocks in rat hippocampal slices. Brain Res 1993; 620: 181–188

[62] Linden DJ. Long-term synaptic depression in the mammalian brain. Neuron 1994; 12: 457–472

[63] Carriere B, Markel FC, Eds. (2006). The pelvic floor. New York: Thieme

[64] Colloca CJ, Keller TS, Harrison DE, Moore RJ, Gunzburg R, Harrison DD. Spinal manipulation force and duration affect vertebral movement and neuromuscular responses. Clin Biomech (Bristol, Avon) 2006; 21: 254–262

[65] Chiu TW, Wright A. To compare the effects of different rates of application of a cervical mobilisation technique on sympathetic outflow to the upper limb in normal subjects. Man Ther 1996; 1: 198–203

[66] McGuiness J, Vicenzino B, Wright A. Influence of a cervical mobilization technique on respiratory and cardiovascular function. Man Ther 1997; 2: 216–220

[67] Sterling M, Jull G, Wright A. Cervical mobilisation: concurrent effects on pain, sympathetic nervous system activity and motor activity. Man Ther 2001; 6: 72–81

[68] Davila GW. Vaginal prolapse: management with nonsurgical techniques. Postgrad Med 1996; 99: 171–176, 181, 184–185

[69] Davila GW, Ghoniem GM, Kapoor DS, Contreras-Ortiz O. Pelvic floor dysfunction management practice patterns: a survey of members of the International Urogynecological Association. Int Urogynecol J Pelvic Floor Dysfunct 2002; 13: 319–325

[70] Davila GW, Guerette N. Current treatment options for female urinary incontinence—a review. Int J Fertil Womens Med 2004; 49: 102–112

[71] Holtzman DA, Petrocco-Napuli KL, Burke JR. Prospective case series on the effects of lumbosacral manipulation on dysmenorrhea. J Manipulative Physiol Ther 2008; 31: 237–246

[72] Proctor ML, Hing W, Johnson TC, Murphy PA. Spinal manipulation for primary and secondary dysmenorrhoea. Cochrane Database Syst Rev 2001 2001;(4): CD002119

[73] Proctor ML, Hing W, Johnson TC, Murphy PA. Spinal manipulation for primary and secondary dysmenorrhoea. Cochrane Database Syst Rev 2004;(3): CD002119

[74] Proctor ML, Hing W, Johnson TC, Murphy PA. Spinal manipulation for primary and secondary dysmenorrhoea. Cochrane Database Syst Rev 2006: CD002119

[75] Maigne JY, Chatellier G, Faou ML, Archambeau M. The treatment of chronic coccydynia with intrarectal manipulation: a randomized controlled study. Spine 2006; 31: E621–E627

[76] Gajeski BL, Kettner NW, Awwad EE, Boesch RJ. Neurofibromatosis type I: clinical and imaging features of Von Recklinghausen's disease. J Manipulative Physiol Ther 2003; 26: 116–127

[77] Martin-Alguacil N, Pfaff DW, Shelley DN, Schober JM. Clitoral sexual arousal: an immunocytochemical and innervation study of the clitoris. BJU Int 2008; 101: 1407–1413

[78] Sbriccoli P, Yousuf K, Kupershtein I et al. Static load repetition is a risk factor in the development of lumbar cumulative musculoskeletal disorder. Spine 2004; 29: 2643–2653

[79] Atiyeh BS. Nonsurgical management of hypertrophic scars: evidence-based therapies, standard practices, and emerging methods. Aesthetic Plast Surg 2007; 31: 468–492, discussion 493–494

[80] Roques C. Massage applied to scars. Wound Repair Regen 2002; 10: 126–128

[81] Roh YS, Cho H, Oh JO, Yoon CJ. Effects of skin rehabilitation massage therapy on pruritus, skin status, and depression in burn survivors. Taehan Kanho Hakhoe Chi 2007; 37: 221–226

[82] Edwards J. (2003). Scar management. Nursing Standard (Royal College of Nursing (Great Britain): 1987), 17(52), 39–42

[83] Frey Law LA, Evans S, Knudtson J, Nus S, Scholl K, Sluka KA. Massage reduces pain perception and hyperalgesia in experimental muscle pain: a randomized, controlled trial. J Pain 2008; 9: 714–721

[84] Herrera I, Ed. (2009). Ending female pain: A woman's manual. New York: Duplex Publishing

[85] Travell JG, Simons DG, Lois LS, Eds. (1999). Myofascial pain and dysfunction: The trigger point manual. Philadelphia, Baltimore, New York, London, Buenos Aires, Hong Kong, Sydney, Tokyo: Lippincott Williams & Wilkins

[86] Cohen SP, Raja SN. Pathogenesis, diagnosis, and treatment of lumbar zygapophysial (facet) joint pain. Anesthesiology 2007; 106: 591–614

[87] Langford CF, Udvari Nagy S, Ghoniem GM. Levator ani trigger point injections: an underutilized treatment for chronic pelvic pain. Neurourol Urodyn 2007; 26: 59–62

6 Treatment

6.1 Introital Pain

6.1.1 Patient Presentation

A patient presents with complaints of introital pain. She is unable to partake in intimate activities that involve vaginal penetration. She states that she is experiencing a progressive loss in tolerance to food due to constipation, and that the stress urinary incontinence that she's been experiencing since the birth of her first child is worsening.

Further questioning reveals that she's had three spontaneous vaginal deliveries (SVDs) —"just pushed them out"—and returned to work as quickly as possible as president of a Fortune 500 company. She had prepared by having a nanny on call. Prior to marriage she had been a nationally ranked figure skater from 8 years old through college, and confirmed the use of oral birth control from the age of 14 to the present, other than to conceive and give birth to her three children.

Treatments to date include Advil, two tablets TID, and self-directed stretching of her "tight pelvic musculature."

6.1.2 Evaluation

- She exhibits extraordinary forward head posture in sitting and standing.
- Her angle of declination is 60 degrees.
- She demonstrates six finger protraction at the scapulothoracic junction.

- ALROM is not provocative for reproduction of patient's symptoms, while there is an apparent decrease of right osteokinematic side-flexion along TL junction.
- Mobility and provocation tests of the sacroiliac joint SIJ are negative.
- She demonstrates a positive prone knee flexion (PKF) on the right, and straight leg raising (SLR) is unremarkable bilaterally.
- Segmental screening for strength and sensation along the L2-S2 nerve roots is unremarkable.
- Increased resting tone throughout the pectoralis minor, sternocleidomastoid, suboccipital group and iliopsoas musculature noted.
- She demonstrates an extraordinary apical respiration pattern.
- Pelvic examination:

  - Upon visual inspection, vaginal inversion is noted where the increased muscle tone of the pelvic floor resulted in the clitoris and anus facing each other
  - Coughing, sneezing, and straining (CSS) were negative
  - Volitional contraction of the pelvic floor musculature (PFM) demonstrates minor lift and slow/modest release; adductor and gluteal accessory contractions noted
  - Upon initiating contact to the ischial tuberosity for the pelvic mapping/palpation, the patient violently withdraws but demands that the evaluation "continue"
  - Bulbospongiosus reflex was negative bilaterally
  - Vaginal sweep was positive for scarring along 11:00 at and along the vaginal-uterine interface
  - Sacral tinel testing was negative
  - Increased tone noted throughout the PFM right > left

6.1.3 Treatment Strategy

In order to best address this patient's pain, where would you initiate your treatment? Complete the listing below, and devise a subsequent treatment strategy for each of the following:
a) Psychology of pain:
b) Neurological considerations:
c) Joint restrictions:
d) Scars:
e) Muscle imbalance and generalized weaknesses:
f) Muscle spasms and fascial restrictions:

In order to address the patient's psychology of pain, she is to be instructed towards the attaining of proper, erect posture. She is to be given means to attain an optimal sitting and standing alignment. McKenzie lumbar support and the like can be introduced. Using a mirror, this patient is to be shown the difference between apical respiration and diaphragmatic respiration patterns. With the use of a mirror, or the supine, book strategy, the patient is to initiate changes in her respiration patterning.

Neurologically, the positive PKF is to be addressed with segmental mobilizations at the T12–L3 junctions. Techniques as outlined in this text, the side-lying rotational mobilizations, or other localized joint specific techniques can be used. After the performance of a joint specific mobilization, the resting tone of the PFM is to be visualized and assessed to determine whether or not there was a change. Many clinicians and patients alike are wonderfully surprised when such a remote treatment has a positive impact on the patient's pain, and resting tone.

Joint restrictions of the thoracic spine are to be segmentally evaluated and treated where they are found. Due to the hyperkyphotic nature described and the predominance of a strong apical respiration pattern, it is very likely that local restrictions will be found.

The scars of the birth canal noted with the vaginal sweep are to be addressed with a gentle transverse friction massage (TFM) (▶ Fig. 6.1). The scar is to be located and gently addressed. If the local pain is significant, consider assessing the thoracolumbar junctions and treating there locally prior to continuing the TFM as the pain may be initiating and enhanced centrally (remember the proximal three-quarters of the internal genital symptoms are conveyed via the hypogastric, pelvic, and vagus nerves to the T5–L2 spinal segments). TFM is to continue at patient's tolerance.

Addressing the patient's muscular imbalance and generalized weakness will involve strengthening of the mid/lower trapezius, the erector spinae, and the abdominal musculature. Examples of these exercises are provided below.

If fascial restrictions persist, the use of ice, in conjunction with the elimination of local joint restrictions, will improve the

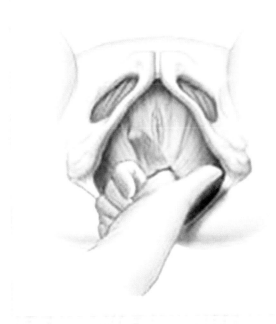

Fig. 6.1 Transverse friction massage.

local mobility. Over the course of the first week of treatment, the clinician and patient alike should notice a marked improvement of local fascial mobility, and improved comfort *if* the patient is actively participating in the postural changes described, and the clinician is providing appropriate joint specific treatments.

6.1.4 Exercises (▶ Fig. 5.13, ▶ Fig. 5.14, ▶ Fig. 5.15, ▶ Fig. 5.16)

The clinician is to progress as is tolerated by each patient. No exercises are to hurt other than typical muscle fatigue and "burn". Pain is to be avoided as pain begets pain. As clinicians we do not want to be a contributor to the enhancement of a patient's pain. Verbal encouragement is often quite necessary and appropriate as those that are suffering are often in poor physical and emotional health.

6.2 Dyspareunia due to SIJ

6.2.1 Patient Presentation

Patient presents with primary complaints of vulvodynia and dyspareunia. She is a 51-year-old woman with a history of two SVDs, 18 and 20 years ago. She denies trauma or a specific event that would have provoked her symptoms. She states that she had gained approximately ten pounds over the past year, and that she finally decided to "take it off." She hired a personal trainer that has her progressing along with her fitness activities. She states that she does not enjoy the workouts, but understands the need to exercise. She reports that the personal training now entails jogging for 1.5 miles and performing a series of box-jumps, *burpies,* and a variety of high-intensity plyometric exercises.

6.2.2 Evaluation

Her symptoms often are noted upon standing from the sitting position, and after standing for more than thirty minutes, along the lumbosacral region with radiations to the groin. She reports a progressive inability to wear high heels as her pain becomes intolerable after fifteen minutes. She further states that she had enjoyed lying on her back on the wooden floor of her apartment to relax, but no longer can tolerate this position due to a progressive building of ache, pain, and distress along the lumbosacral region. She states that her right more so then her left buttock is hurting; spasms are present.

When she attempts to be intimately active, she experiences pain upon penetration, but that external contact and clitoral stimulation are normal. She has greater tolerance to penetration while in the rear-entry position, while her preferred position (missionary position) is becoming intolerable.

She finds herself thinking frequently about her pain, and often digitally "checks" her pain during bathroom breaks to see if she is tolerating vaginal penetration on any given day. To her dismay, she is tolerating digital contact and penetration less and less each day.

- Patient stands with an angle of declination of 65 degrees bilaterally.
- Patient demonstrates five finger protraction bilaterally at the scapulothoracic joint (STJ).

- ALROM is unremarkable other then an absence of lumbar lordosis reversal in full flexion.
- Myotomal/dermatomal screening of lumbosacral nerves is unremarkable.
- Gillet and standing flexion tests were positive on the right.
- Neural tension testing of the sciatic nerve is unremarkable.
- Prone knee flexion test is provocative for pain at the right > left SIJ; positive Nachlas test.

  ○ When the hip is extended, and the prone knee flexion maneuver is performed, the pain is more pronounced at the ipsilateral SIJ; Yeoman's test.
- SIJ compression is mildly provocative on the right, negative on the left for local symptoms along the SIJ, while SIJ decompression is alleviating of vulvodynia symptoms.
- ASLR is unremarkable.
- FABER, FAIR, McCarthy and tests for the posterior labrum are unremarkable.
- When the hip is flexed, adducted toward the contralateral coxofemoral hip and then an axial pressure is exerted through the femur, the patient complains of her inguinal/vulvodynia pain right > left.

  ○ Stressing iliolumbar ligament
- Positive "Dead Butt Syndrome" findings right > left.

Clinical question: would you perform an internal pelvic examination at this time? If so, what clinical indications do you have to justify the progression of the evaluation? If not, why would you choose not to perform an internal evaluation as she has a history of two SVDs, and penetration dyspareunia?

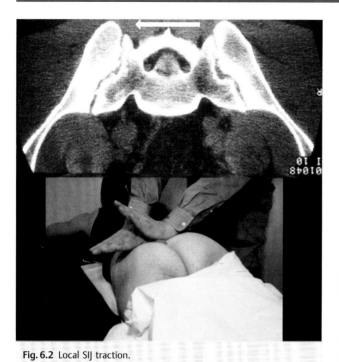

Fig. 6.2 Local SIJ traction.

6.2.3 Treatment Strategy

In order to best address this patient's pain, where would you initiate your treatment? Complete the listing below, and devise a subsequent treatment strategy for each of the following:
a) Psychology of pain:
b) Neurological considerations:
c) Joint restrictions:
d) Scars:
e) Muscle imbalance and generalized weaknesses:
f) Muscle spasms and fascial restrictions:

Psychology of pain: the patient is to be advised and encouraged to avoid the persistent self-evaluation and perseveration over her vaginal penetration pain. Constant attention thereto will enhance her local pain due to the activation of the RVM/PAG, and with repeated noxious stimulation to the region she unknowingly will enhance her pain via central and peripheral sensitization.

Neurological considerations: The prone knee flexion was positive, but the patient's reported symptoms were along the SIJ ipsilaterally, and the symptoms increased with hip extension. This process indicates more involvement of the SIJ then the femoral nerve. This, coupled with the positive Gillet and standing flexion tests, a reduction of symptoms during SIJ decompression, and stress testing of the iliolumbar ligament, indicate a great likelihood of SIJ involvement. The Dead-Butt syndrome findings further indicate local involvement of the SIJ. The coxofemoral joint and related structures appear to be unremarkable. Treatment is to be initiated at the right SIJ. Local transverse friction massage to the iliolumbar ligament, followed by a local SIJ traction and mobilization to the SIJ as outlined by Grieves offered the patient great relief of her vulvodynia pain (▶ Fig. 6.2).

Scars: There were no scars noted, but crepitus was noted along iliolumbar ligament.

6.2.4 Exercises

Muscle imbalances are then addressed and include exercises as indicated in ▶ Fig. 5.9, ▶ Fig. 5.10, ▶ Fig. 5.11, ▶ Fig. 5.12.

At the end of treatment, an internal evaluation was never conducted. The patient had full return of comfort during intimate and non-intimate activities. Reminder: the SIJ can refer pain anteriorly, and with perseveration, local pain and dysfunction can be enhanced. She was given strengthening activities and postural education to ensure healing and full wellness.

6.3 Sign of the Buttock

6.3.1 Patient Presentation

Consider the patient that presents himself with considerable pain along the left gluteal region. Sitting is intolerable, so he sits with his weight shifted heavily to the right. Upon questioning the patient states that he'd been mountain biking when his front tire locked and he was catapulted over the top of his handlebars, landing on his left buttock. He has a significant past medical history involving the L5 intervertebral disc, and recalls having buttock pain that was similar, but less intense than he is presently experiencing.

6.3.2 Evaluation

Upon inspection, the patient can barely flex forward as his pain is extraordinary. When taken to supine, as standing was no longer tolerated, straight leg raising was positive on the left and the symptoms worsened with passive hip flexion with knee flexed.

The evaluation concluded immediately, and the patient was taken to a local hospital. Why?

The field of physical therapy is evolving and we as practitioners are often becoming the "gatekeepers" for a patient's pain and dysfunction. We, as professionals, must always keep in mind that serious pathology does occur, and in this case, the patient had a dislocated sacral fracture.

6.4 Labral Tear

6.4.1 Patient Presentation

Patient is seen status-post left labral repair of the hip. Conservative care and restoration of motion and functional strength progress properly and the patient is fully capable of returning to 80% of her prior activities without limitations as it relates to her hip. She does, however, continue to complain of ipsilateral inguinal pain, and pain that is reported to be "deep" to the buttock ipsilaterally.

6.4.2 Evaluation

Clinical examination:

• The lumbar spine is clear, unremarkable.
• The SIJ is clear, unremarkable.

- While supine, with hips flexed, the clinician palpates medial to the ischial tuberosity pressing the palpating digit in a cranial and lateral oblique angle and the patient remarks that there is considerable pain all the while the clinician notes crepitis under the palpating digits.
- After performing a transverse friction massage via pronation and supination of the forearm the patient notices a considerable decrease of her pain. At follow-up visit, the patient reports that the pain had subsided for the remainder of the day, but returned upon waking the next day. This procedure of TFM was repeated for the subsequent two visits with similar results.

6.4.3 Treatment Strategy

In order to best address this patient's pain, where would you initiate your treatment? Complete the listing below, and devise a subsequent treatment strategy for each of the following:
a) Psychology of pain:
b) Neurological considerations:
c) Joint restrictions:
d) Scars:
e) Muscle imbalance and generalized weaknesses:
f) Muscle spasms and fascial restrictions:

Psychology of pain: The patient did not exhibit any signs or symptoms of perseveration.

Neurological considerations: No tests were found to indicate neurological involvement.

Joint restrictions: Upon healing from the surgery, there were no local joint restrictions noted.

Scars: Palpation of the obturator internus, externally, provided two significant findings: One, crepitus to palpation that was associated with the patient's pain reproduction, and two, local treatment thereto alleviated the patient's symptoms. The progression of treatment involved the performance of an internal evaluation of the obturator internus and pelvic structures. This revealed a protective spasm of the obturator internus and after local treatment thereto the patient demonstrated full, pain-free motion of the hip.

6.5 Plantar Fasciitis

6.5.1 Patient Presentation

A 40-year-old woman presents with persistent medial heel and plantar fascial pain. She states that she is unable to walk without wearing sneakers, and that the pain upon initially stepping out of bed is at least a 9/10. Slow walking will reduce the pain, but after any rest, her initial steps are extremely painful. She has custom and over-the-counter orthotics, to no avail. She stretches daily. She has worn the "boot" for six months straight at night, to no avail. She has endured local deep tissue massage to the plantarfascia, posterior tibialis and "every" muscle of the foot and ankle.

The patient has a history of three SVDs with episiotomy. She denies a loss of bladder or bowel function. She does report "tightness" in the posterior thigh after intercourse in the missionary position, but attributes this to age and a general lack of fitness.

6.5.2 Evaluation

Lumbar evaluation was negative for motion, or segmental testing of the dermatomes from L2–S1. She demonstrated a positive Gillet tTest and a positive jump test for the left sacroiliac joint, indicating local hypomobility, while local stress tests were negative.

After discussing the sacral nerves and anterior SIJ ligaments, and the option to evaluate these via internal evaluation, the patient agreed to an evaluation. During the course of the internal evaluation the following were noted:

- decreased tone and relative bulk of the right pubovaginalis and rectalis; apparent avulsion from the pubis
- scarring throughout the muscle belly of the pubovaginalis and rectalis
- pain with crepitus along the left anterior SIJ ligament
- reproduction of patients right heel and posterior thigh pain with Tinel testing of the S2 and S3 nerve roots respectively

6.5.3 Treatment Strategy

In order to best address this patient's pain, where would you initiate your treatment? Complete the listing below, and devise a subsequent treatment strategy for each of the following:
a) Psychology of pain:
b) Neurological considerations:
c) Joint restrictions:
d) Scars:
e) Muscle imbalance and generalized weaknesses:
f) Muscle spasms and fascial restrictions:

Psychology of pain: The patient did not exhibit any signs or symptoms of perseveration.

Neurological considerations: The presence of a positive Tinel testing along the S2/3 nerve roots indicates local irritation thereto. The clinician must then determine why these nerve roots are irritated, and then make a determination of how they are to address this irritant. For this patient, the findings of local left SIJ hypomobility strongly indicated that local treatment thereto would be appropriate. This, however, would be limited in success if the right-sided weakness as a result of the breach in the pubovaginalis and rectalis were not also addressed. Inlay the balance between treating the neurological considerations, while keeping in mind the body-as-a-whole. In order to adequately address the neurological findings, I chose to mobilize the left SIJ with the local traction and Grieve's SIJ mobilization. This was followed by transverse friction massage to the right sided pubovaginalis and rectalis.

As the local motion of the SIJ improved, and the tissue quality improved of the pubovaginalis and rectalis, I was able to introduce local strengthening thereto. As had been conducted during the evaluation outlined previously, the splitfinger assessment of the PFM indicated right-sided weakness. Local resistance to the pubovaginalis and rectalis allowed for a re-strengthening of the musculature. Much like treatments to partial tears of the rotator cuff or quadriceps muscle, re-union of the torn musculature is not to be expected from a physical therapists treatment capacity. Functional strengthening of the remaining tissue, however, is frequently possible and best achieved after the local scarring has been eliminated.

With strengthening of the PFM, the patient was then taken through a series of progressive strengthening activities that include traditional table/plinth exercises with internal palpation (to ensure use of musculature), and progressed to standing/closed kinetic chain exercises (including free-standing squatting, and various yoga poses inclusive of the Warrior series) to attain full functional stabilization of the SIJ. The result was an elimination of stresses placed on the S2/3 nerve roots and an elimination of her "plantarfascial" pain.

6.6 Central Sensitization/ Embryologic Derivation of Pain

6.6.1 Patient Presentation

A 50-year-old man presents with complaints of severe pain at the tip of his penis. He states that it is as if "1,000 knives" are stabbing him continually. He reports that he is unable to sit without this pain magnifying considerably. He further continues that he has been unable to work and was subsequently terminated from his otherwise successful career as an attorney in a local law firm. He was projected to make partner in the firm in a year's time, prior to his termination. His house is currently in foreclosure, and his wife of ten years has filed for divorce as a direct result of his inability to make love to her (due to the pain in his penis) and their financial constraints as a result of his vocational termination. With further questioning, he reports a progression of his pain to include the right testicle. He feels as if it is being compressed in a vise, and that the pressure increases as the day "drags on" daily, each day worse than the previous.

6.6.2 Evaluation

Clinical observation: He sits in the most contorted, kyphotic position imaginable. Pressure primarily through his right lateral hip/pelvis, and a striking left rotation of the shoulder/chest is noted. In standing he presents with a seven digit protraction of the right shoulder blade, and five of the left. His lower cervical spine is painfully flexed and flattend, while that of the upper cervical spine is hyper extended. The thoracic hyperkyphosis is so extreme that there are callous formations along the spinous processes of T9–L1. Respiration is labored and apical. He has a recent history of arthroscopic removal of his gallbladder as a result of digestive "issues" that he'd previously suffered.

Clinical evaluation demonstrates poor active motions of the lumbar and thoracic spine, with an inability to extend the lumbar spine beyond neutral, and left side-flexion of the thoracic and lumbar spines are limited to a few degrees. Right rotation of the thoracic spine is five degrees, while that of left rotation is fifteen. Inspection of the ribs demonstrates a protraction and hypomobility of the 10th rib on the right. Segmental testing of the lumbar myotomes and dermatomes is insignificant. Segmental motion of the spine indicate an absence of motion at the T9–12 segments; local fulcrum of motion at L1/2.

Pelvic observation: The testes and the penis are withdrawn dramatically, resembling that of an enlarged vagina, more so than that of a male appendage. The perineum and anus demonstrate a sustained lift, and local muscle twitches can be visualized. The patient insists that you perform an internal evaluation "to rid him of this disastrous disease," yet he yelps in agony with contact to the ischial tuberosity while initiating the pelvic mapping palpation outlined previously. Pelvic palpation and evaluation was discontinued at this point.

6.6.3 Treatment Strategy

In order to best address this patient's pain, where would you initiate your treatment? Complete the listing below, and devise a subsequent treatment strategy for each of the following:
a) Psychology of pain:
b) Neurological considerations:
c) Joint restrictions:
d) Scars:
e) Muscle imbalance and generalized weaknesses:
f) Muscle spasms and fascial restrictions:

Psychology of pain: This gentleman attributes a significant portion of his recent "failures" to be directly related to his pain —loss of work, loss of house, and loss of his marriage.

Segmental mobilizations in right side lying of the T9–T12 segments was initiated at a grade of I and II; T10/11 segments are the common embryological derivation for the gall bladder, epididymis, and penis. Postural education provided, and the 10th rib was addressed via a posterior–lateral mobilization at the sternum; 10th rib adversely impacts function of gall bladder. Ice was used along the T9–12 segments, and diaphragmatic education and home exercises were introduced.

Very slow therapeutic exercises consisting of hip abduction, adduction, extension, and quad setting were initially introduced so as to allow successful reintegration of exercises without regression or perceived regression. These movements were coupled with education towards appropriate diaphragmatic respiration during exercises. Postural education was introduced, and demonstrated in a mirror with the patient to assist in the awareness of what a neutral spine looks like and feels like. As he slowly gained underlying muscle strength and coordination, the therapeutic exercises were progressed to include latissimus dorsi pull downs and rows, traditional abdominal crunches, and light aerobic exercises on the treadmill and stationary bicycle.

6.7 Peripheral Sensitization/ Bladder Dysfunction

6.7.1 Patient Presentation

Patient presents with a primary complaint of urgency of the bladder. She has the tell-tale key lock phenomenon whereupon opening the front door of her house, she has the extraordinary need to find the bathroom to release her "full" bladder. This phenomenon is occurring more frequently and intensely at home, and within the past month at work. She finds herself needing to use the bathroom hourly, sometimes more frequently. Her sleep is interrupted, and complains of extraordinary fatigue, and is concerned that she may be jeopardizing her career as her productivity is noticeably decreasing due to the frequent trips to the bathroom.

6.7.2 Evaluation

She has a history of two SVDs, 4 and 8 years previously. She denies significant bladder dysfunction after the first month of having given birth on both occasions. She confirms that she "Kegels" daily, and the more sensitive her bladder has become, the more she "Kegels."

She denies pain during ADLs, and confirms that her sex life is "good" and without pain. She does admit, however, that she seems to have lost the ability to attain an orgasm, but is confident that this is due to an overall exhaustion in lieu of having two active children, a full-time job, and interrupted sleep.

Evaluation of the lumbar spine is unremarkable, other than right-sided positive prone knee flexion and point tenderness over the pubic symphysis; positive crepitus. SIJ distraction/pubic symphysis compression is provocative, while SIJ compression/pubic symphysis distraction examination is reported as "relieving."

Pelvic examination demonstrated minor vaginal gapping with minor bulge upon coughing; negative leakage. Upon request there was a notable lift, with minimal hiatal closure. External palpation was negative, other than episiotomy scarring at 7 o'clock. Layers one, two, and three manual muscle testing demonstrated a 2/5 on the right, and 3/5 on the left. The vaginal sweep indicated scarring of the pubovaginalis and a remarkable loss of muscle bulk from 9 o'clock to 12 o'clock (at the pubis). Palpation of the urethra demonstrates a leftward angulation, with irritable fine crepitus along the left side thereto, and globular, course crepitus along the right side of the urethra. The bulbospongiosus reflex was hyporeactive on the right side, while normal on the left. Tinel testing of the sacral and pudendal nerves was unremarkable.

6.7.3 Treatment Strategy

In order to best address this patient's pain, where would you initiate your treatment? Complete the listing below, and devise a subsequent treatment strategy for each of the following:
a) Psychology of pain:
b) Neurological considerations:
c) Joint restrictions:
d) Scars:
e) Muscle imbalance and generalized weaknesses:
f) Muscle spasms and fascial restrictions:

Psychology of pain: The patient demonstrated no signs of cognitive dysfunction.

Neurological considerations: The patient demonstrated a hyproreflexive right bulbospongiosus reflex, *and* a mechanical breach of the right-sided pelvic floor musculature. In the absence of SIJ testing being positive, it is very likely that the apparent retardation of the reflex may be reflective of the musculature breach, more so than a nerve root compromise. The findings of right-sided prone knee flexion indicate involvement of the (L1)/L2/3 nerve roots, both of which provide sensory innervation to the anterior pubic symphysis. From an embryological perspective, the bladder has a T11, 12, and L1 origin, and the urethra is S2, 3, 4, and 5.

Joint restrictions: Immediate attention and treatment was directed at L1 and L2. This provided alleviation of not only the bladder sensitivity but also of that along the urethra. Why so? Due to the process of peripheral sensitization, the persistent irritability along the bladder due to pubic symphysis irritation led to an expansion of the receptor field to include the urethra. Therefore, treatment of urethral symptoms was attained via treatment at segments of the spine that is otherwise unrelated to the urethra.

Transverse friction massage was provided to bilateral urethra, the sphincter urethra, and the right side pubovaginalis.

The muscle imbalance was addressed by use of manual resistance to the right side of the pelvic floor musculature, and this patient demonstrated a restoration of bulk along the remaining portions of the pubovaginalis that had otherwise not been noted/palpable initially due to the degree of atrophy prior to strengthening. The patient was taught how to facilitate strengthening of the pelvic floor musculature with an internal digit providing greater facilitation/resistance to the right pelvic floor.

6.8 Torn pubovaginalis leading to increased use of pubococcygeus, fecal retention.

6.8.1 Patient Presentation

A 50-year-old woman presents with complaints of fecal retention. She states that she feels a progressive bulging within the vagina simultaneously as the rectum pressure progresses. She states that intimacy is often initially uncomfortable but tolerable, and progresses to comfortable. She continues to states that she often places a digit vaginally to assist in the evacuation of the bowel, and that during the more difficult bowel movements she must manually evacuate the rectum using a gloved hand/finger. She admits to having surgical gloves in her purse "all the time."

6.8.2 Evaluation

Her history includes three SVDs with grade III fissures to the anus left. Negative loss of urine other than during coughing episodes while ill.

Lumbar evaluation is negative other than an angle of declination of 65 degrees, and crepitus along bilateral SIJ.

Pelvic examination demonstrates a bulge along the posterior vaginal hiatus that increases with volitional contraction of the pelvic floor musculature. There is minimal lift noted. Moderate labial separation noted at rest, increasing with contraction of PFM. External palpation is unremarkable for pain. Separation of the labia minora demonstrates the presence of the distal bowel distending the vaginal canal, occupying more than half the orifice. Upon palpation, it moves easily out of the way, but immediately returns to its fallen/resting position upon release.

Assessment of the PFM indicates significant tone along the posterior margin of the vaginal hiatus and minimal tone along the lateral aspects of the vaginal wall. Layer-to-layer evaluation of the PFM indicates poor overall capacity to contract the first layer of musculature bilaterally, while the second layer was noted to be symmetrical at 3 + /5. The third layer demonstrated 3-/5 on the right, while the left was 1/5. There was an absence of bulk throughout the left side of the PFM originating immediately posterior to the pubis, just lateral to the symphysis, while approximately one finger's breadth lateral thereto is appropriate bulk, albeit with extraordinary tautness, tenderness, and crepitus. Palpation of the anterior SIJ ligament demonstrated course crepitus bilaterally, and Tinel testing of the sacral and pudendal nerves was unremarkable.

6.8.3 Treatment Strategy

In order to best address this patient's pain, where would you initiate your treatment? Complete the listing below, and devise a subsequent treatment strategy for each of the following:
a) Psychology of pain:
b) Neurological considerations:
c) Joint restrictions:
d) Scars:
e) Muscle imbalance and generalized weaknesses:
f) Muscle spasms and fascial restrictions:

Psychology of pain: The patient is apparently coping, and dealing well with her condition.

Neurological findings were modest. The weakness noted is likely due to the breach of musculature along the left pubovaginalis and the distension of the distal bowel into the vagina, blocking muscle activity. While this is the working assumption, if her strength doesn't improve, then further neural evaluation is to be conducted and treated as necessary.

Joint restrictions: Sustained central posterior to anterior (CPA) pressure at S3 were conducted both with and without the use of a pelvic floor contraction to assist in a counternutation of the sacrum.

Scars: The scars along the length and origin of the pubovaginalis were addressed with a transverse friction massage. With activation of the pelvic floor musculature, and after the performance of the aforementioned mobilizations, it was found that the remaining fibers of the pubovaginalis responded and hypertrophied over the first three weeks. Local points of scar, denoted via palpation of crepitus, continued to be addressed via transverse friction massage.

The muscle weakness and asymmetry of the pubovaginalis was addressed with manual resistance with a palpating digit. Initially, a stretch facilitation was required. This progressed along well, and to my wonderful surprise, there was a relative restoration of relative bulk and nearly (95%) symmetrical strength.

6.9 Conclusion

The purpose of this textbook is to examine the concepts of differential diagnosis and to apply them to the patient with pelvic pain. To do so, a thorough review of the multitude of structures involved with the initiation, perpetuation, and expansion of pelvic pain is discussed so that the clinician can understand and determine what treatment techniques are to be applied to best address the origin of the patient's pain. When practiced properly, the clinician can expect to make immediate changes in the patient's well-being, and with proper progression of education, and exercises, these changes can be permanent.

There are no "cookbook" answers to a patients' pain. Clinicians must learn to accurately determine the initiating and perpetuating aspects of a patient's pain presentation to most efficiently manage symptoms and provide the patient the opportunity to heal.

Study hard, work hard, and have great success!

Index